Silencing Migraines

A Survivor's Guide

By
Dr. Felix Fielding

Silencing Migraines

A Survivor's Guide

Table of Contents

Introduction

Migraines, a condition that affects millions globally, often present a daunting challenge. For the unacquainted, they're not just headaches. They're a complex neurological ailment that can disrupt lives in profound ways. This unpredictability and intensity can lead sufferers down a path of frustration, isolation, and seeking elusive relief. But it doesn't have to be a path walked alone or in darkness. Empowerment comes through understanding and effective management strategies, which are central to finding ease and navigating life with migraines.

This book is born from a need to untangle the complexities surrounding migraines. It's not just for those who suffer but also for friends, family, and healthcare providers who stand in support. Our goal is simple yet profound: to impart knowledge that aids in the practical management of this condition. Through this lens, we discuss the unique experiences of migraine sufferers, exploring how they can regain control and enhance their quality of life. It is about shifting from enduring migraines to actively managing them.

In exploring migraines, one quickly discovers there is no universal experience. The throbbing at the temples for one individual might be an aura-induced visual disturbance for another. For some, migraines are sporadic, hinted at by discernible triggers like certain foods or stress. For others, they linger in a chronic state, becoming a more significant feature in the backdrop of life. This book acknowledges these varied experiences while seeking to provide a comprehensive guide that speaks to all.

Our journey begins with understanding what migraines truly are and the science that explains them. This knowledge forms the foundation from which you can build practical solutions. With insight into potential triggers, readers can begin to decipher their unique migraine signatures, laying the groundwork for the strategies and adjustments detailed in subsequent chapters.

But understanding alone is insufficient. Effective management calls for action across multiple fronts—lifestyle changes, dietary considerations, and mental well-being are all vital components. By modifying daily routines and stress management techniques, many have found an unexpected degree of relief. Coupled with dietary adjustments, the path to migraine management becomes clearer and more manageable. It's about making informed decisions that align with one's lifestyle and needs.

Medical treatments also play a crucial role. Staying informed about the latest over-the-counter and prescription options is imperative. Similarly, alternative therapies offer additional avenues for relief, with practices like acupuncture and the use of herbal supplements gaining traction. This book aims to illuminate the benefits and potential pitfalls of various treatments and therapies, always prioritizing safety and efficacy.

Beyond physical symptoms, the emotional toll of migraines is unquantifiable. This book gives due attention to coping strategies and the importance of emotional support. We're here to discuss pain management techniques that go beyond medication, to include emotional resilience and building a strong support network. It's about creating a toolkit of practices that fortify one's emotional state against the stresses of living with migraines.

Tracking and analyzing patterns through migraine journals is encouraged throughout our discussion. Such records can illuminate triggers and helpful interventions, offering a clearer picture over time. Collaborating with healthcare professionals becomes all the more effective when combined with comprehensive records, enriching the dialogue and enhancing the pursuit of relief.

Social dynamics can be another arena where migraines exert influence. Whether navigating social situations, explaining symptoms to friends and family, or managing migraines in the workplace, effective communication and preparation are key topics we tackle. Understanding how to articulate one's needs, while securing necessary accommodations, transforms potentially isolating experiences into opportunities for support and understanding.

As migraines ebb and flow, packing up for a trip can become another chapter fraught with concern. Not anymore. Equipped with travel tips tailored to their needs, migraine sufferers can explore the world with more confidence and less anxiety. The emphasis here is on planning and the adaptability that enables sufferers to engage with life fully, despite the unpredictability of their condition.

Moreover, the relationship between sleep and migraines, hormonal fluctuations for some, debunking common myths, and the perplexing world of chronic migraines lend themselves to deeper exploration. These factors are intrinsic to the pathology of migraines and are addressed thoroughly, ensuring readers have a holistic understanding.

As we move through patient stories and case studies, this book paints a mosaic of lived experiences. These narratives serve to connect, inform, and inspire, providing both solace and strategy. Readers can glean wisdom from others who have traveled similar roads, learning about techniques and solutions that have proven effective in managing migraines over the long term.

Ultimately, the empowerment journey we embark on in this book isn't just about finding relief from pain. It's about reclaiming one's life. It's about discovering ways to thrive in the face of adversity, understanding the interplay of mind and body, and finding solidarity in a community of shared experiences. For that, this book is your companion, your atlas guiding you through the multifaceted world of migraines, reminding you at every step that while migraines are complex, the pursuit of relief doesn't have to be walked alone.

Chapter 1:
Understanding Migraines

Migraines are more than just headaches; they are a complex neurological condition that affects millions of people worldwide, causing debilitating pain and a host of other symptoms. Understanding migraines involves exploring the intricate science of how they originate in the brain, including the complex interplay of genetic and environmental factors. It's crucial to recognize that migraines vary significantly from person to person, not only in terms of triggers but also in their frequency, duration, and intensity. While some might experience aura, others may endure nausea or heightened sensitivity to light and sound. By delving into the intricacies of migraines, sufferers and their loved ones can begin to identify patterns and triggers unique to their experiences, paving the way for more personalized and effective management strategies.

The Science Behind Migraines

Migraines are more than just severe headaches. At their core, they represent a complex neurological condition marked by recurring episodes of painful headaches, often coupled with a host of other symptoms. To truly grasp the science behind migraines, it's essential to understand the genetic, biochemical, and physiological elements that contribute to their onset and progression.

One of the foundational theories explaining migraines is the role of the central nervous system's hyper-excitability. Essentially, an individual with migraines may have a brain that responds excessively to certain stimuli, leading to a cascade of neurological activities that culminate in migraine attacks. This hyper-reactivity is believed to be influenced by genetic factors, with research showing that migraines often run in families. Studies have identified several genes associated with familial migraine patterns, suggesting a hereditary component.

At a molecular level, migraines appear to be linked to the neurotransmitter serotonin and its receptors. During a migraine attack, levels of serotonin fluctuate significantly, causing the blood vessels in the brain to constrict and then dilate. This change in blood vessel diameter is associated with the throbbing pain that many migraine sufferers experience. Moreover, specific genetic mutations affecting ion receptors in the brain have been linked to disruptions in normal serotonin function, further implicating this pathway in the pathophysiology of migraines.

Beyond serotonin, another critical component in the science behind migraines is the trigeminovascular system, which involves the trigeminal nerve. This nerve is a major pain pathway within the brain. When triggered, it releases pro-inflammatory neuropeptides, including calcitonin gene-related peptide (CGRP), which leads to inflammation and pain. Behavioral and environmental factors can excessively activate this system in migraine sufferers, further exacerbating symptoms.

Technological advancements in the field of neuroimaging have provided incredible insights into what happens in the brain during a migraine attack. Utilizing MRI and other imaging techniques, researchers have observed a phenomenon known as cortical spreading depression, a wave of electrophysiological activity that moves across the brain's cortex. This wave is associated with changes in blood flow, which can precipitate the aura experienced by some migraine sufferers—a series of sensory disruptions that often precede the headache phase.

Aura, commonly experienced as visual disturbances or tingling sensations, offers clues about the brain's involvement in migraine onset. Thought to result from a short period of reduced cortical activity, followed by an increase, aura underlines how migraines affect both the brain's function and its vasculature.

Another layer to consider in understanding migraines is the role of the hypothalamus. Positioned deep within the brain, the hypothalamus is responsible for regulating various bodily rhythms, including sleep, hunger, and hormonal output. Dysfunction in these areas is often reported by individuals experiencing migraines. Migraines often manifest cyclically, suggesting the hypothalamus could serve as a trigger point for these attacks, influencing hormonal cycles and the body's internal clock.

Genetic predisposition, coupled with external stimuli, informs the diversity of triggers for migraines. Researchers suggest a complex interplay between genetic and environmental factors. External triggers like stress, certain foods, or changes in weather can activate the migraine cascade in those predisposed genetically. However, the precise mechanism by which these triggers affect the nervous system remains a subject of ongoing research.

Investigation into hormonal influences offers further insights into the science of migraines. Notably, the prevalence of migraines is higher in women than men, which has led scientists to explore the role of sex hormones, particularly estrogen. Fluctuations in hormone levels, often occurring during menstrual cycles, pregnancy, and menopause, have been closely linked to migraine frequency and intensity. Understanding these dynamics underscores the importance of tailored treatment approaches that consider both biological and hormonal factors.

In summary, the science behind migraines is a mosaic of numerous interconnected factors. There's a unifying theme that encompasses genetic predispositions, neurotransmitter imbalances, involved neural circuits, hormonal influences, and external triggers. As ongoing research continues to unravel these complexities, the promise of more targeted and effective treatments for migraine sufferers becomes more tangible. With each breakthrough, we move a step closer to demystifying this enigmatic condition, offering hope for improved management and, eventually, more effective solutions for those affected by migraines.

Common Triggers

Migraines are a complex neurological condition, and understanding the everyday factors that can lead to an attack is crucial in managing them effectively. For those who experience migraines, identifying specific triggers is often the first step toward relief. Yet, it's a challenging task, as these triggers can vary significantly from one person to another.

One of the most prevalent triggers is stress. In today's fast-paced world, stress is an unavoidable part of life. It can arise from various sources, such as work, family obligations, or even positive life changes. The link between stress and migraines is strong, as stress can lead to changes in brain chemicals, impacting the body and potentially triggering a migraine.

Environmental factors can also play a substantial role. Bright or flickering lights, strong odors, and loud noises are commonly reported migraine triggers. These sensory inputs can overstimulate the brain, causing it to react in ways that lead to a headache. For some, just a few minutes in a bright or noisy environment is enough to provoke an attack.

Weather changes are another frequent—and frustrating—trigger. Shifts in barometric pressure, as well as extreme heat or cold, can spur a migraine. Individuals sensitive to these changes may find that their migraines correlate with stormy weather or seasonal transitions. Unfortunately, avoiding weather-related triggers can be impossible, making other management strategies even more vital.

Hormonal changes are particularly significant for many migraine sufferers, especially women. The fluctuation of hormones, such as estrogen, during menstrual cycles, pregnancy, and menopause, can either trigger or exacerbate migraine attacks. Tracking hormonal patterns and their impact on migraines often helps in predicting and managing these occurrences.

Dietary triggers are another significant category. For many, specific foods and beverages can provoke a migraine. Common culprits include alcohol, particularly red wine, caffeine, and foods containing additives like MSG and artificial sweeteners. Keeping a food diary can help individuals pinpoint problem foods and understand their body's responses.

Sleep patterns also hold the keys to migraine onset. Both too little and too much sleep can trigger an attack. Irregular sleeping schedules, interrupted sleep, or poor sleep quality can disturb the brain's balance, making consistent sleep patterns essential for migraine management.

Dehydration is a simple yet often overlooked trigger. Not drinking enough fluids can lead to headaches, making staying hydrated crucial. For those prone to migraines, particularly during exercise or hot weather, increasing water intake can be a preventive measure.

Beyond these individual triggers, it's important to recognize that migraines are often the result of cumulative factors. One trigger alone may not be enough, but a combination of stress, dietary choices, and environmental exposures might lead to an attack.

Understanding these triggers provides valuable insights for migraine sufferers. By identifying and avoiding known triggers where possible, individuals can reduce the frequency and severity of their migraines. With careful observation and documentation, one can discern patterns that might otherwise go unnoticed.

While recognizing triggers is vital, it's just the beginning. Developing a comprehensive plan that addresses these triggers is key to managing migraines effectively. This often involves lifestyle adjustments, dietary changes, and stress management techniques.

Moreover, sharing trigger patterns with healthcare providers can lead to more personalized treatment plans. A nuanced understanding of one's triggers can also assist in reducing medication reliance by focusing on prevention rather than just treatment.

The journey to managing migraines involves patience, persistence, and a willingness to learn from both triumphs and setbacks. With knowledge and proactive strategies, one can navigate the complexities of migraines, ultimately leading to better days and a healthier life. By embracing this understanding of common triggers, migraine sufferers empower themselves on the path to lasting relief and improved quality of life.

Chapter 2:
Diagnosing Your Migraine

Understanding your migraine's unique patterns is crucial for effective management, as it allows you to identify specific triggers and seek the most appropriate treatments. Often, migraines are accompanied by a variety of symptoms that can vary widely among sufferers. Recognizing these signs early on can lead you to more insightful discussions with your healthcare provider, who plays a pivotal role in your migraine journey. As you work together, they'll guide you through various diagnostic tools and tests, helping to paint a clearer picture of your condition. This collaborative approach not only validates your experiences but also empowers you with the knowledge to anticipate and mitigate future attacks. By investing time in this diagnostic phase, you lay the foundation for informed decisions and a proactive path toward relief and recovery.

Identifying Symptoms

Recognizing the symptoms of migraines is the first step toward gaining control over this often debilitating condition. While each individual's experience with migraines can vary significantly, there are common threads in the patterns and types of symptoms that sufferers may encounter. It's essential to unravel these threads to achieve a clearer understanding of what a migraine truly entails.

Initially, many people will find themselves struggling to differentiate between a typical headache and a migraine. The key lies in the intensity and accompanying features. Migraines are often more severe, accompanied by a throbbing or pulsating pain, usually on one side of the head. The pain can intensify with physical activity, light, sound, and sometimes specific smells, setting migraines apart from the usual headache. By acknowledging these distinct features, one can begin to identify their condition as more than just "a bad headache."

Migraine symptoms can be broken down into four stages, though not everyone experiences all stages. These stages are prodrome, aura, headache, and postdrome. Understanding these phases can help sufferers and healthcare professionals develop a more nuanced approach to diagnosis and treatment. They also offer insight into what to expect and when, allowing individuals to prepare and manage their symptoms more effectively.

In the prodrome phase, subtle changes such as mood swings, food cravings, neck stiffness, or increased thirst might occur. These symptoms can begin a day or two before the onset of the migraine itself. Recognizing these early warning signs can be an empowering skill, enabling one to take preemptive measures like resting or adjusting daily activities to mitigate the impact of the impending migraine.

The aura phase, experienced by about 25% of migraine sufferers, presents a more dramatic array of symptoms, often happening before or during the headache. Auras are typically visual disturbances like seeing flashes of light or zigzag patterns. Some might experience tingling in the limbs or face, difficulty speaking, or even temporary vision loss. These experiences can be unsettling but are crucial indicators that a migraine is looming.

Moving to the headache phase, the hallmark symptom is the aforementioned intense, throbbing head pain. This pain is frequently accompanied by nausea, vomiting, or heightened sensitivity to light and sound. This stage can last from a few hours to several days, severely impacting a person's quality of life and ability to perform everyday tasks.

After the headache subsides, the postdrome phase can create a feeling of exhaustion and confusion, akin to a "migraine hangover." During this time, sudden head movements might briefly cause pain. It's a recovery stage where the body is recalibrating, and energy levels often feel depleted. Taking it easy during this phase is crucial, as pushing oneself could trigger another episode.

Additionally, migraines sometimes present as more than just head pain. Some individuals experience abdominal pain, especially younger sufferers, termed as abdominal migraines. These can involve serious digestive symptoms and might not involve a headache at all, making diagnosis tricky but essential for proper management.

Despite these general categorizations, symptoms can be idiosyncratic, presenting unique challenges in diagnosis. For instance, silent migraines occur without head pain, focusing instead on other symptoms like aura or nausea. Such variations highlight the importance of personalized medical approaches and attentive symptom tracking.

Symptoms can also be influenced by external factors and personal health conditions. Hormonal changes, particularly in women, play a significant role and often influence the timing and severity of migraines. This aspect will be covered in detail in the section on "Hormones and Migraines," but it's important to note here as it underscores the variability and complexity of migraine symptoms.

Understanding these symptoms within the broader context of one's lifestyle and health can be profoundly beneficial. By tracking the onset, duration, and type of symptoms, individuals can gain insights into potential triggers, which are yet another critical aspect of migraine management discussed further in "Common Triggers." A proactive approach is not just about recognizing symptoms but utilizing that understanding to reduce the frequency and intensity of future episodes.

Ultimately, the journey of identifying symptoms is deeply personal. It requires patience and careful observation. But beyond simply identifying the markers of a migraine, this knowledge serves as a foundational tool in the overarching goal of managing and reducing the impact of this condition, thus improving life quality for anyone dealing with migraines.

Working with Healthcare Providers

When it comes to diagnosing migraines, a partnership with healthcare providers is indispensable. Establishing a solid relationship with your doctor can lead to a more accurate diagnosis and effective management plan. This relationship is a collaborative effort that involves clear communication, trust, and a commitment to exploring various avenues of treatment.

It all starts with choosing the right healthcare provider. Not every doctor specializes in migraines, so it's beneficial to seek out a neurologist or a headache specialist. These professionals have a deeper understanding of the nuances involved in migraine diagnoses and can offer more targeted treatment options. A good place to begin your search is through recommendations from your primary care physician, or by consulting resources provided by migraine support organizations.

Once you've found a suitable healthcare provider, the key is to be as detailed and forthcoming as possible about your symptoms. Migraines can manifest in a multitude of ways, and the more information you can provide, the better. This means noting the frequency, duration, and intensity of your headaches. Do you experience nausea, sensitivity to light, or visual disturbances? No detail is too small.

Keeping a migraine diary can be incredibly beneficial in this process. It assists not only in tracking symptoms but also in identifying potential triggers and patterns over time. Share this valuable resource with your healthcare provider during consultations. Together, you can pinpoint elements that might be contributing to your migraines, leading to more tailored advice and treatment plans.

Open communication with your healthcare provider also entails discussing your current treatment regimen and any other medications you're taking. Be sure to mention over-the-counter drugs you frequently use, as these can sometimes contribute to rebound headaches or interact with prescription medications. Transparency is pivotal to avoiding complications and finding the most effective path forward.

As you work with your healthcare provider, don't hesitate to ask questions or seek clarification. It's entirely appropriate to inquire about the rationale behind suggested treatments or tests, as understanding your care is crucial to empowering yourself in the management of your condition. Be informed about potential side effects, expected outcomes, and alternative strategies should the initial plan prove ineffective.

Sometimes, despite the best efforts, a treatment may not yield the desired results. This is where patience and persistence come into play. It may take some time to find the right combination of treatments that work for you. It's not uncommon to try several approaches before discovering what best alleviates your symptoms. This trial-and-error process should be viewed as a journey that both you and your healthcare provider navigate together.

It's also vital to stay abreast of new developments in migraine research and treatment options. New therapies and medications are continuously being developed. Engaging in discussions about these innovations during appointments can open doors to cutting-edge treatments that you may not have considered before.

If at any point you feel dissatisfied with your care or the progression of your treatment plan, it's completely appropriate to seek a second opinion. Another healthcare provider might offer fresh perspectives or alternative approaches that better suit your needs. Your comfort and confidence in your healthcare team are paramount.

Working with healthcare providers isn't just about appointments and prescriptions; it's about building a supportive network that includes you as a key player. Over time, you'll become more than a passive recipient of healthcare; you'll transform into an empowered individual who actively participates in managing migraines.

And don't forget, healthcare providers extend beyond doctors. Pharmacists, therapists, dietitians, and alternative medicine practitioners can play crucial roles in holistic migraine management. For instance, a dietitian might help optimize your nutrition, while a therapist could support your mental well-being in dealing with chronic pain.

Your healthcare provider can also guide you in incorporating non-medicinal therapies into your routine. These might include cognitive-behavioral therapy, yoga, or stress reduction techniques, all of which can serve as powerful complements to more traditional treatments.

As the landscape of healthcare evolves, telemedicine has become an invaluable tool. Virtual consultations provide a flexible and convenient way to maintain regular contact with your healthcare provider—a game changer for those whose migraines might make traveling to appointments challenging.

Finally, remember that mutual respect is the foundation of any successful partnership. Just as you rely on your healthcare provider for expertise and guidance, they rely on your honesty and commitment to the treatment plan. This mutual understanding fosters an atmosphere where innovative solutions thrive, and better health outcomes become more attainable.

By actively engaging with your healthcare providers and leveraging their expertise, you'll be well equipped to navigate the complexities of migraine diagnosis and management with greater confidence and efficacy. Together, you can turn the tide on migraine's debilitating effects, creating a life that is not just about managing pain, but enhancing wellness and empowerment.

Chapter 3:
Lifestyle Adjustments

As we transition into addressing lifestyle adjustments, consider how nuanced yet powerful these changes can be in the journey of managing migraines. Integrating mindful modifications into daily life serves as a cornerstone for reducing the frequency and intensity of headaches. Establishing a consistent daily routine, prioritizing quality sleep, and making time for relaxation are pivotal steps towards fostering a migraine-resilient lifestyle. The subtle art of listening to your body's signals embodies a proactive stance, turning potential triggers into opportunities for proactive care. With determination and adaptability, lifestyle changes hold the promise of significant relief, reminding us that the path to wellness often starts with the choices we make every day.

Daily Routine Changes

For those navigating the relentless world of migraines, adjusting daily routines can be a transformative stride toward relief. The cornerstone of managing migraines lies in understanding that seemingly trivial day-to-day activities often wield significant influence over one's migraine threshold. Migraines can be tenacious adversaries in the battle for normalcy, but they don't have to dictate every moment. By carefully crafting and adhering to a routine tailored to the individual's needs, the impact of migraines can be lessened, ultimately enhancing one's quality of life.

Adopting consistency is perhaps the most potent weapon in this personal arsenal. Consistency in sleep, meals, exercise, and overall daily schedules can significantly lower the frequency and severity of migraine attacks. While change is an inevitable part of life, striving for stability in day-to-day timings can help establish a rhythm that the body responds to positively. Such consistency isn't just about routine but about cultivating a lifestyle that gently nurtures the mind and body, providing them with the reliable cues they crave.

Let's begin with something as fundamental as the morning routine. Waking up at the same time each day can greatly contribute to a sense of balance. This routine gives your internal clock the signal it needs to promote a steady circadian rhythm. Equally important is allowing yourself a gentle start to the day. Introducing a few minutes for light stretching or deep breathing exercises can set a positive tone, easing you into what lies ahead without sudden jolts to your system.

Breakfast, often dubbed the most important meal of the day, doubles as a cornerstone in migraine management. Skipping meals or delaying eating can act as a trigger for migraines. Therefore, it's crucial to prioritize a nutritious breakfast that incorporates protein, healthy fats, and complex carbohydrates. This balance helps to maintain blood sugar levels, reducing the likelihood of triggering a migraine. Building this habit of mindful eating starts the day right and equips the body with sustained energy.

The workday presents its own set of challenges and opportunities for routine optimization. Regular breaks are essential, especially when working at a desk or using digital screens. Every 30 to 60 minutes, take a moment to stand up, stretch, and walk around, even if just for a couple of minutes. This doesn't only relieve physical tension but also provides a mental reset, reducing stress levels and subsequently cutting down migraine risk. Consider integrating moments of mindfulness throughout the day, brief check-ins with oneself to assess how they're feeling physically and mentally.

Hydration plays a critical role in staving off migraines. Dehydration is a common trigger that can easily be avoided by ensuring a steady intake of water throughout the day. Having a water bottle at hand serves as a constant reminder to stay hydrated. While caffeine intake can be a double-edged sword, it's necessary to understand your own body's response to it and use that knowledge to your advantage. Some may find that moderate caffeine intake can alleviate migraines; for others, it may act as a catalyst if consumed excessively.

Another pivotal aspect of routine adjustment involves task management and organization. Stress and anxiety can be potent triggers, and often, they're exacerbated by feeling overwhelmed. Breaking down tasks into manageable segments and prioritizing responsibilities can ease this sense of overwhelm. Each small completion engenders a sense of achievement and control, which can be empowering and reduce stress-related migraine triggers.

As the day winds down, preparing the body for restful sleep is crucial. Establishing a predictable bedtime routine can aid in signaling to the brain that it's time to relax. This process might include avoiding screens at least an hour before bed, engaging in relaxing activities like reading or taking a warm bath, and ensuring the sleeping environment is conducive to rest; dim lighting and comfortable temperatures support this goal. These steps will be examined in more detail in the section focused on the importance of sleep.

On weekends or days off, it might be tempting to deviate from regular routines, but such variations can provoke migraines in those sensitive to change. Striking a balance between allowing oneself a break and maintaining consistency where possible is key. Planning leisurely activities that still align with overall routine objectives, such as scheduling meals and keeping similar sleep timings, helps mitigate risk.

Integrating these changes is not about restriction but rather about finding freedom within boundaries. It's about redefining one's relationship with routine as a source of predictability amidst life's unpredictabilities. By implementing thoughtful daily adjustments, those living with migraines can cultivate an existence marked by empowerment rather than constraint, turning each day into a canvas for better managing their condition.

Importance of Sleep

Migraines have a way of crashing into our lives, uninvited and unpredictable. For those battling these relentless headaches, sleep can either be a trusted ally or a potential foe, depending on its quality and consistency. The relationship between sleep and migraines is deeply intertwined, underscoring why establishing and maintaining a healthy sleep schedule is pivotal for managing migraines effectively.

Let's begin by acknowledging the power of restorative sleep. Quality sleep nurtures the brain, restores energy, and rejuvenates the body. It's not merely the hours we accumulate under layers of blankets but the depth and uninterrupted nature of our sleep cycles that contribute to its restorative potential. Missing out on these nourishing hours can lead to a restless mind and a body on edge, setting a fertile ground for migraines to flourish.

Intrinsically linked to our circadian rhythms, which regulate our sleep-wake cycles, disturbances in sleep can directly impact the frequency and intensity of migraine episodes. A regular, predictable sleep cycle can foster stability in the brain's complex network of electrical impulses and prevent the deviations that might trigger migraines. Many migraine sufferers find that even modest disruptions—late nights, early mornings, or inconsistent routines—

can upset this delicate balance, often resulting in increased vulnerability to migraine attacks.

The journey to better sleep—and consequently better migraine management—often begins with simple yet profound changes in lifestyle. Establishing a consistent sleep and wake schedule is the bedrock of improved sleep hygiene. When your body gets accustomed to a regular rhythm, it can prepare itself physiologically for when to sleep and when to wake, reducing the chances of lagged or disrupted sleep that can trigger migraines.

Let's delve deeper into the mechanics of sleep to further understand its importance in managing migraines. During a typical sleep cycle, the body progresses through a series of stages, from light sleep to deeper, more restorative REM sleep. These stages are essential for various physiological processes, including hormone regulation and emotional processing. It's during REM sleep that the brain becomes particularly active, and this phase is crucial for memory consolidation and mood stabilization.

Moreover, achieving higher quality sleep can aid in minimizing the stress levels that often accompany migraines. Stress is a well-known migraine trigger, and those suffering from migraines often find themselves trapped in a vicious cycle—where migraines induce stress, which in turn could lead to more frequent migraines. Sleep has a critical role in breaking this cycle. When we sleep, our bodies undergo physiological processes that lower stress hormones, allowing our minds a much-needed respite from daily stresses.

However, the reality for many migraine sufferers is that sleep itself can sometimes feel elusive, a paradoxical companion that's hard to attain. Anxiety about impending migraines might lead to sleep problems, which, in turn, exacerbate the migraines. It becomes imperative to approach sleep as a strategic aspect of migraine management, employing practical methods geared towards improving sleep quality.

There's an arsenal of tools and techniques that can enhance sleep quality, thereby minimizing migraine episodes. Creating a sleep-friendly environment is fundamental. This entails optimizing your surroundings to be as conducive to rest as possible. Consider dimming the lights in the evening and using blackout curtains to keep distractions to a minimum. Cultivating such an environment encourages the natural production of melatonin, a hormone that helps regulate sleep.

Another effective strategy is practicing relaxation techniques before bed. Techniques such as progressive muscle relaxation or mindful breathing can pave the way for a smooth transition from daytime activities to restful slumber. These methods help in decreasing anxiety and activating the body's natural relaxation response, making it easier to drift off to sleep.

Electronics, while indispensable in our modern lives, can disrupt sleep with their blue light emissions which interfere with melatonin production. Limiting screen time an hour before bed, or using apps that filter blue light, can help safeguard your sleep quality. It's also worth considering keeping a regular bedtime routine, including activities such as reading or listening to calming music, to signal to your body that it's time to wind down.

Dietary considerations can also play a role in sleep quality and should be taken into account. Caffeine, alcohol, and large meals before bedtime can impact the ability to fall and stay asleep. Reducing the intake of these substances, particularly in the hours leading up to sleep, can significantly enhance the sleep experience.

For those struggling with more persistent sleep issues, professional support can offer vital insights. Consulting with sleep specialists or cognitive-behavioral therapy for insomnia (CBT-I) practitioners can unravel more deeply ingrained sleep issues and offer structured guidance on creating tailored sleep strategies. Professional interventions can provide a pathway to understanding and resolving underlying issues that may be contributing to poor sleep and, by extension, frequent migraines.

Ultimately, recognizing the immense benefits of quality sleep is a vital step for anyone coping with migraines. By adopting a proactive approach towards better sleep, individuals can cultivate a lifestyle that supports both their neurological health and overall well-being. As part of a comprehensive lifestyle adjustment, prioritizing sleep isn't just about clocking more hours in bed—it's about embracing the restorative power of sleep to lead a healthier, more balanced life free of migraines' grasping influence.

Chapter 4:
Dietary Considerations

Navigating the intricate landscape of dietary considerations is pivotal in managing migraines, as the food we consume wields significant influence over our neurological functions. Understanding that certain foods can provoke a migraine while others offer relief empowers those afflicted to make informed choices that can potentially diminish the frequency and intensity of these debilitating episodes. It's not just about avoidance; identifying beneficial nutrients that support brain health and enhance well-being can become a beacon of hope. Each person's triggers vary, yet arming oneself with knowledge of general dietary patterns that have shown promise can foster a sense of control and optimism. As we delve deeper, embracing a diet that nurtures rather than hinders could symbolize a major turning point in the journey toward a more balanced, pain-free life.

Foods to Avoid

Understanding the connection between diet and migraines is crucial for anyone looking to manage their symptoms effectively. While every individual might respond differently to specific foods, certain dietary patterns and components have been identified as common culprits in triggering migraines. Knowing what to avoid can empower migraine sufferers, providing them with a clearer path to better health and symptom management.

One of the most well-documented triggers is processed meats, such as bacon, hot dogs, and deli meats. These are often high in nitrates and nitrites, preservatives that can dilate blood vessels and possibly trigger migraines. Interestingly, the same nitrates that preserve the meats' bright pink hue can also spark the painful neural pathways associated with migraines. It's advised to limit consumption or seek nitrate-free alternatives.

Beyond processed meats, certain cheeses are notorious for causing headaches—usually those that are aged. Cheese varieties like cheddar, blue cheese, and parmesan contain tyramine, a substance known to cause migraines in some individuals. Tyramine forms as the protein in cheese breaks down over time, hence the higher levels in aged cheeses. Keeping a food diary can help determine if these cheeses are a personal trigger.

Chocolate, a beloved comfort food, can unfortunately be a migraine trigger for some. It contains both caffeine and beta-phenylethylamine, potential culprits in the onset of migraines. While not everyone will react to chocolate, those who notice an association between consuming this treat and migraine onset should consider moderation or alternative snacks.

Speaking of caffeine, it's a double-edged sword in migraine management. While small amounts might help alleviate headaches, excessive caffeine intake or sudden withdrawal can induce migraines. The key is consistency—if you're a coffee drinker, try to keep your daily intake steady and be cautious about abrupt changes in your caffeine routine.

Avoiding artificial sweeteners, particularly aspartame, is another tip to keep in mind. Used widely in diet sodas and sugar-free products, aspartame might trigger migraines in sensitive individuals. The exact mechanism isn't fully understood, but the anecdotal evidence and some clinical observations suggest that replacing these sweeteners with natural alternatives could be helpful.

Alcohol, especially red wine, ranks high on the list of dietary triggers. It's rich in tannins and sulfites, both of which might trigger migraines in susceptible individuals. The dehydrating properties of alcohol can also contribute to headaches. For many, limiting alcohol or choosing carefully is a prudent approach.

Next, consider MSG (monosodium glutamate), a flavor enhancer frequently used in processed foods and some Asian cuisine. MSG might provoke migraines by affecting neurotransmitters or through direct effects on blood vessel dilation. Checking ingredient lists and opting for MSG-free products can be beneficial.

It's important to note that citrus fruits, while generally healthy, might induce migraines in some people. The underlying reason may be related to fluctuations in acidity levels or certain compounds that spark nerve sensitivity. Experimenting with citrus intake and observing any changes in headache patterns could provide valuable insights.

Bread and baked goods made with yeast might also lead to migraines. The fermentation process in yeast can produce tyramine, one of the notorious headache triggers. Identifying yeast-containing foods and watching their influence on your migraine symptoms is a helpful strategy.

Last but not least, soy products, including soy sauce, tofu, and some meat substitutes, contain both tyramine and MSG in varying amounts. These can be hidden triggers lurking in seemingly innocuous meals. It's worthwhile to examine food labels and opt for alternatives if you notice a correlation.

As with any dietary advice, personalization is key. Each person's response to food triggers can be unique; what ignites a migraine in one person might be perfectly safe for another. Keeping a migraine diary that tracks food intake and symptoms can be a transformative tool. It provides insights not only on what to avoid but also on the overall relationship between diet and migraine health. In this journey, knowledge is power—and understanding dietary triggers can significantly reduce the frequency and intensity of migraines, improving quality of life.

Beneficial Nutrients

The journey to understanding how diet influences migraines often unveils the power of beneficial nutrients in managing these debilitating headaches. Among the many dietary considerations that can help reduce the frequency or severity of migraines, certain nutrients stand out for their potential impact. Integrating these nutrients into your diet can serve as a game-changer, not just mitigating symptoms but also enhancing overall health.

Magnesium is one such nutrient that has garnered attention for its role in migraine relief. It's involved in numerous bodily functions, including nerve transmission and muscle contraction, both of which can affect migraine dynamics. Studies have shown that people who suffer from migraines often have lower levels of magnesium. Hence, incorporating magnesium-rich foods like spinach, almonds, and dark chocolate may provide much-needed relief.

Another nutrient worth noting is riboflavin, or vitamin B2. Known for its capacity to boost energy production in brain cells, riboflavin has been linked to reduced migraine frequency. Leafy greens, eggs, and dairy products are excellent sources of riboflavin, making them valuable additions to a migraine-friendly diet.

Omega-3 fatty acids are also vital, given their anti-inflammatory properties. Found abundantly in fatty fish like salmon, flaxseeds, and walnuts, omega-3s can help decrease the frequency and intensity of migraine attacks by modulating inflammatory responses in the body.

Regular consumption of omega-3-rich foods can also support cardiovascular health, making them an all-around excellent choice.

Coenzyme Q10 (CoQ10) is another player in the field of migraine management. This antioxidant is essential for cell energy production and has been associated with reduced migraine frequency. While it's available in foods like organ meats and whole grains, supplementation might be necessary to achieve therapeutic levels. Consulting with a healthcare provider before beginning any supplement regimen is advisable.

In the realm of vitamins, vitamin D's role in migraine relief is gaining recognition. Known for its involvement in maintaining bone health and immune function, vitamin D deficiency has been observed in many migraine sufferers. Sunlight is a primary source, but fortified foods and supplements can help maintain adequate levels, especially during months with limited sun exposure.

The discussion of beneficial nutrients wouldn't be complete without mentioning hydration. While not a nutrient in itself, water intake is critical. Dehydration is a well-recognized trigger for migraines, and maintaining hydration status can significantly impact the frequency and severity of attacks. Emphasizing water-rich foods like cucumbers and watermelons can help meet daily hydration needs.

There's also evidence pointing to the benefits of ginger, particularly its anti-inflammatory and anti-nausea properties. Sipping on ginger tea or adding freshly grated ginger to meals may alleviate some migraine symptoms, providing a natural and palatable method of relief.

When discussing diet and nutrients, it's crucial to recognize that individual responses can vary. What works remarkably well for one person might have minimal effects on another. Keeping a food and symptom diary can help identify personal triggers and beneficial foods, leading to more tailored dietary adjustments.

Navigating the world of nutrition can feel overwhelming, particularly for those prone to migraines. Yet, by focusing on incorporating these beneficial nutrients, there's promise for decreasing the burden of headaches and improving overall quality of life. The journey to wellness is deeply personal, and paying attention to how one's diet influences migraine patterns is a vital step in the process.

If dietary interventions are new territory, it may be helpful to work alongside a nutritionist or a healthcare provider familiar with migraines to develop a personalized nutrition plan. This strategy allows for professional guidance tailored to your specific needs, ensuring a balanced intake of these beneficial nutrients while considering any other health concerns.

In conclusion, the path to reducing the frequency and intensity of migraines may very well start with what's on your plate. By consciously integrating nutrient-rich foods into your diet, you're taking significant strides toward migraine management and optimal health. Always remember your health is an evolving journey, and every positive change, no matter how small, brings you closer to a life with more clarity and fewer headaches.

Chapter 5:
Stress Management

Life's challenges can easily send stress levels spiraling, yet managing stress is crucial in navigating the turbulent waters of migraine management. It's no secret that stress acts like a trigger for these relentless headaches, but taking control is not as daunting as it might seem. By integrating effective stress management techniques into your daily routine, you're not just reducing the frequency and severity of migraine attacks, but also enhancing your overall well-being. Start small with simple relaxation practices—like deep breathing or listening to calming music. Add mindfulness and meditation to your toolkit, as both can ground you in the present moment, helping your mind break free from perpetual cycles of worry. Embrace these strategies as lifelines, ensuring they fit snugly into your lifestyle, and gradually watch as their impact unfolds. Take the reins of stress, and in doing so, reclaim a portion of your life dominated by migraines. As you do, remember you are not alone; countless others have walked this path and emerged resilient, hopeful, and perhaps even inspired to live life more fully despite the challenges.

Relaxation Techniques

In the quest for relief from migraines, relaxation techniques emerge as a beacon of hope. They offer not just a short respite but a path to long-term serenity. Anyone who's ever been gripped by a migraine knows the overwhelming tension that precedes and accompanies the pain.

While it's not the sole solution, relaxation can significantly reduce the frequency and intensity of headaches. Let's delve into some effective methods that can be seamlessly integrated into daily life.

The first step in adopting relaxation techniques is creating an environment that fosters peace. Picture this: a quiet, dimly-lit room, perhaps enhanced by calming scents like lavender or chamomile. The idea is to disengage from stress triggers and provide your mind with a sensory escape. Just spending ten minutes in such an environment can clear away incessant thoughts and ease physical tension.

Deep Breathing is one of the most accessible relaxation methods. It's free and can be performed almost anywhere. By focusing on slow, deep inhalations, followed by deliberate exhalations, you encourage the body to release tension. The physiological impact is significant: deep breathing lowers heart rate and blood pressure, giving the body a signal to relax. In times of stress, many tend to breathe shallowly, which can exacerbate migraine symptoms. Deep breathing exercises can counteract this by introducing a sense of calm and control.

Visualize yourself by the ocean, listening to waves lap at the shore. This type of *guided visualization* can be remarkably effective. It involves painting a mental image of a tranquil scene, integrating all senses to make the visualization as vivid as possible. It distracts from pain and fosters a mindful state, promoting relaxation and reducing migraine severity.

Progressive Muscle Relaxation (PMR) is another potent technique. This involves systematically tensing and then relaxing different muscle groups in the body. The contrast between tension and relaxation heightens awareness of physical stressors, aiding in the release of residual muscle tightness often prevalent during migraines. With practice, sufferers can identify areas of tension and consciously release them, reducing the onset of a migraine.

Integrating technology, *biofeedback* devices serve to train individuals to gain control over physiological functions they might not typically engage with consciously. These devices display data regarding stress markers like heart rate and skin temperature. With this information, users learn to harness techniques like controlled breathing or meditative practices to reduce stress levels, contributing to migraine relief.

Yoga and Qi Gong offer holistic approaches. These disciplines combine physical postures with breathing exercises, promoting a profound state of relaxation. The gentle movements and emphasis on breath control help reduce stress hormones, improve circulation, and enhance overall well-being, often resulting in fewer migraine episodes.

The power of **music therapy** should not be underestimated. Soothing melodies can lower anxiety, a significant migraine trigger. Playing calm, rhythmic music creates a tranquil ambiance, encouraging a release of tension throughout the body. Music's rhythmic nature aids in stabilizing the mind's heartbeat, much like how ocean waves might calm an anxious night.

Meditation presents itself as an essential tool in managing stress. It's more than a practice; it's a shift in consciousness. By fostering a state of reflective stillness, meditation enables the mind to focus away from pain. It cultivates awareness and acceptance, providing a safe space away from the discomfort of migraines. Regular meditation nurtures resilience, acting as a buffer against stressful situations that might otherwise trigger headaches.

Journaling can also be a therapeutic exercise; it offers an emotional outlet to release pent-up frustrations. By writing down worries and stresses, you create a narrative that can be externalized, analyzed, and subsequently addressed. This act of confronting stressors on paper diminishes their power, unraveling emotional knots that might contribute to headaches.

Finally, consider nurturing *positive social interactions*. Sharing thoughts with trusted friends or family members can significantly alleviate feelings of loneliness or anxiety. Engaging in lighthearted conversation or participating in fun activities provides mental distraction, balancing cortisol levels and promoting relaxation.

While no single technique is a panacea, incorporating a combination into daily routines fosters an atmosphere conducive to relaxation. Consistency is key, as even a brief regular practice can yield substantial benefits. Empowerment through relaxation is a journey, one where you'll uncover resilience and fortitude, discovering little by little how much power you truly possess over your migraines. These serene moments break the cycle of relentless tension, guiding you toward a world where pain loses its grip.

Mindfulness and Meditation

In the midst of the daily pressures and frantic pace of modern life, the gentle embrace of mindfulness and meditation can serve as a sanctuary for those grappling with migraines. There's an undeniable power in pausing and bringing one's awareness to the present moment, a power that's been increasingly recognized in managing stress-related aspects of migraines. These practices aren't just about silence or sitting still; they are about cultivating an acute awareness and a deep, compassionate engagement with the mind and body.

Meditation, in its many forms, has been a cornerstone of wellness for centuries, deeply rooted in ancient traditions across cultures. Whether practiced through focused attention, loving-kindness meditation, or body scan methods, it offers a spectrum of approaches that can be tailored to suit individual needs and conditions. For migraine sufferers, the very nature of meditation as a tool for relaxation can help in lowering stress, which is often a key trigger for episodes.

Mindfulness, a term that has become almost ubiquitous in wellness conversations, is more than a trendy buzzword. It's a mental state achieved by focusing one's awareness on the present moment, routinely through meditation, while calmly acknowledging and accepting one's feelings, thoughts, and bodily sensations. For individuals with migraines, this acceptance and non-judgmental observation can alleviate some of the anticipatory anxiety that often accompanies the condition. By learning to acknowledge pain non-reactively, sufferers may experience a shift in how they perceive their discomfort.

Scientific studies have begun to illuminate the neural mechanisms behind why mindfulness and meditation are effective. When one meditates, there's evidence suggesting that the brain experiences a reduction in activity in the default mode network (DMN), the area responsible for mind-wandering and self-referential thoughts. Less activity in the DMN can lead to a quieter mind, which in turn may reduce the brain's hypersensitivity to pain stimuli—a common problem for those with migraines. Moreover, regular practice of mindfulness and meditation can enhance emotional regulation, providing sufferers with a valuable tool to combat the mood disturbances often intertwined with chronic pain.

For those just beginning to explore these practices, the journey need not be daunting. You don't need a dedicated meditation room or lengthy sessions to start seeing benefits. Consider starting with short, guided sessions that can be as brief as five minutes. Numerous apps and online resources provide accessible entry points, offering a plethora of guided meditations tailored specifically for stress relief and pain management. Over time, these brief meditations can become more intuitive, eventually integrating seamlessly into daily life.

Incorporating mindfulness into everyday activities can also be transformative. This practice doesn't require additional hours in the day; it's about finding moments of presence amidst the ordinary. Whether it's during a morning walk, while savoring a meal, or even in the act of brushing your teeth, these instances can become opportunities to practice mindfulness. Notice the sensations of each step, the flavors and textures of the food, the rhythm of the brush against your teeth. Each moment of mindfulness is a moment less governed by stress, anxiety, and pain.

The holistic benefits of these practices extend beyond the mind. There is growing evidence that mindfulness and meditation can also lead to physiological changes, such as lowered blood pressure and reduced levels of the stress hormone cortisol. These changes can contribute to a reduction in the frequency and intensity of migraine attacks, providing a compelling argument for their inclusion in a comprehensive migraine management plan.

Connecting with the breath is another fundamental aspect of both mindfulness and meditation. When a migraine begins to rear its head, turning to a few minutes of focused breathing can be a powerful tool to calm the nervous system. Breathing deeply, slowly, and deliberately can help shift the state of your body from one of stress and tension to one of relaxation and ease. This simple yet profound act gets you back in touch with your body, allowing you to gently guide it away from an episode prompted by heightened stress or anxiety.

To fully reap the benefits of mindfulness and meditation, consistency is vital. Mindfulness is a skill, one that requires practice and patience to cultivate. Integrating these practices as a regular part of life can be a challenge at first, but with persistence, the ease and presence they bring can shift from a fleeting experience to a new way of being. Keep in mind that there is no "right" way to practice meditation or mindfulness. Everyone's journey is unique, and what works for one might not work for another. It's about finding what resonates most and trusting that process.

In closing, as you embark on or continue this journey of self-care through mindfulness and meditation, remember that it's not about eradicating all pain but rather transforming your relationship with it. It's about fostering a state of ease in the midst of discomfort and finding peace even when confronted by the storm of migraines. In doing so, you'll not only take vital steps towards managing your migraines but also enrich your overall quality of life, offering yourself grace, patience, and understanding along the way.

Chapter 6:
Exercise and Physical Activity

Incorporating exercise and physical activity into your routine can be a powerful tool in managing migraines. While the idea of working out might seem daunting, especially when headaches loom, research shows that regular physical activity can lead to significant improvements in overall health and migraine frequency. Exercise releases endorphins, which act as natural painkillers, and helps reduce stress, a common migraine trigger. The key lies in moderation and finding activities that don't exacerbate your symptoms—gentle exercises like yoga, tai chi, or walking can be incredibly beneficial. By gradually building up your endurance and listening to your body's cues, you can transform exercise into an empowering part of your migraine management plan. Remember, it's about discovering what works best for you and integrating movement in a way that enhances, rather than hinders, your journey to wellness.

Safe Exercises for Migraine Sufferers

Finding the right types of exercise can be pivotal for those battling migraines. As anyone who suffers from migraines knows, physical exertion sometimes becomes both a relief and a trigger. This paradox can leave people feeling hesitant about incorporating activity into their routines. However, by choosing the right exercises and understanding their bodies' signals, migraine sufferers can embrace physical activity to enhance their well-being.

Low-impact exercises can offer substantial benefits without the risk of exacerbating migraine symptoms. Activities like walking, swimming, and cycling tend to be gentle on the body. They're ideal for maintaining cardiovascular health, improving circulation, and reducing stress—all of which can contribute to fewer and less-intense migraine episodes. A 30-minute daily walk, particularly in a peaceful setting, might provide both physical benefits and a calming mental respite.

Swimming is another excellent choice. It provides a full-body workout that's easy on the joints and muscles. The buoyancy of water can soothe the body and help dissipate tension. If you're near a body of water or pool, consider integrating swimming into your routine. Start with short sessions and gradually increase the duration as you gauge your comfort and response.

It's crucial to listen to your body. Awareness of how you're feeling during and after exercise can help prevent migraine triggers. A consistent and gentle approach is best. If you sense a migraine approaching, it might be wise to stop activity and rest. Hydration is essential too. Dehydration can be a significant trigger, so ensure you're drinking plenty of water before, during, and after physical activity.

Mindful exercises, such as yoga and tai chi, blend physical movement and mental stillness, focusing on balance, flexibility, and controlled breathing. These practices not only strengthen muscles and enhance posture but also encourage relaxation and stress reduction. Yoga, in particular, has been noted for its calming effects on the nervous system, which might help reduce migraine frequency and severity. Gentle poses can be modified to fit an individual's comfort level, ensuring that even those with restricted mobility can participate.

Before embarking on a new exercise regimen, consult with a healthcare provider. They can offer personalized advice based on your medical history and specific needs. A physician familiar with your migraine history will likely recommend starting slowly and progressively increasing intensity based on your tolerance.

It's also beneficial to complement exercise with relaxation techniques. Using tools like guided imagery or deep-breathing exercises during cooldowns can enhance the migraine-moderating benefits of physical activity. By interlinking these strategies, one can create a holistic approach to managing migraines, reducing the potential for attacks triggered by overexertion.

Incorporating regular aerobic exercise helps maintain a healthy weight, further reducing the risk of migraines. This is not just about aesthetics; a healthy body weight is directly correlated with the frequency and severity of migraine episodes. Endorphins released during moderate exercise act as natural pain relievers, potentially decreasing the reliance on medication.

If possible, find an exercise buddy. Having someone to walk with or join you in a yoga class adds a layer of social support, motivation, and accountability. Sharing the journey with someone can make activities more enjoyable and rewarding, especially on days when the motivation might wane.

While sunshine and fresh air can be invigorating, for migraine sufferers, they can sometimes trigger symptoms. If you're exercising outdoors, consider timing your activities to avoid the sun's peak hours or using protective gear like hats and sunglasses. Indoor alternatives can be just as rewarding. Gyms, home workout videos, or even walking indoors on days when the environment seems unfriendly to your health are all viable options.

Balancing exercise intensity with migraine triggers can be a challenge, but it's not insurmountable. Understanding your body and working with it, rather than against it, aids in not just migraine management but also in fostering a healthier lifestyle. The key is consistency and the willingness to adapt based on what your body tells you.

Ultimately, no single exercise regimen works universally; it's about discovering what feels right and beneficial for you. Remember, the goal is to empower yourself with the knowledge and tools needed to manage migraines effectively, integrating exercise as a complementary component of your overall health strategy. Acknowledging the nuances of migraine experiences, there's hope and capacity to live a vibrant life, empowered by movement and mindful living strategies.

Benefits of Regular Activity

It's easy to overlook the benefits of regular physical activity when a migraine strikes. The pounding headache, the nausea, and the aversion to the brightest corners of any room seem to scream, "Rest is what's needed!" Yet, regular exercise is not just about shedding pounds or building muscle; it's a compass pointing towards wellness, gently nudging us away from the throes of chronic headaches.

Firstly, let's talk endorphins. These little neurotransmitters, often dubbed the body's natural painkillers, are released in the brain through physical activity. From a brisk walk in the park to a gentle yoga session, exercise can increase endorphin production, helping to stave off the perception of pain. For those battling migraines, these chemicals can make a substantial difference.

Beyond endorphins, regular exercise helps modulate some of the underlying causes of migraines. The stress response, a common trigger, can be significantly dampened through physical activity. Exercise reduces levels of the body's stress hormones, such as adrenaline and cortisol, and, in turn, lowers overall stress levels.

Let's not forget about the importance of blood circulation. Consistent aerobic exercise enhances blood flow to all parts of the body, including the brain, where migraines often wreak the most havoc. Improved circulation ensures that the brain receives a steady supply of oxygen and nutrients, which could help prevent the onset of migraines.

Regular physical activity also promotes better sleep – a boon for migraine sufferers who know firsthand how lack of quality rest can provoke an attack. Exercise can help regulate your sleep cycle, making it easier to fall and stay asleep, ensuring you wake up refreshed and less susceptible to migraines.

Moreover, exercise offers a powerful tool to manage weight, which is of particular interest to migraine sufferers. Research shows a link between obesity and increased frequency and severity of migraines. By incorporating physical activity into your routine, managing weight becomes more feasible, potentially reducing the frequency and intensity of migraine episodes.

It's worth noting, too, that exercise cultivates a sense of empowerment and control. When you're dealing with the often unpredictable nature of migraines, having a kind of go-to practice—a run, a swim, or even a series of tai chi movements—can provide a sense of routine and stability amidst the chaos.

While the advantages of regular activity are clear, it's important to approach exercise with caution and awareness. Start slow and choose activities that feel comfortable, particularly when in the midst of migraine symptoms. Low-impact exercises, like walking, biking, or swimming, are often recommended.

Staying consistent with physical activity can also serve as a form of preventive care. This isn't just about slashing acute symptoms—it's about long-term strategy. When exercise becomes a part of daily living, it reinforces a lifestyle which marginalizes migraines.

Furthermore, exercise can enhance mood levels, which is vital for those wrestling not only with migraines but the accompanying emotional strain. It's well-documented that physical activity, through the release of endorphins, can alleviate feelings of depression and anxiety—conditions frequently associated with chronic headaches.

Considering the holistic benefits, regular exercise harmonizes with other lifestyle modifications discussed throughout this book. Whether paired with dietary changes, stress management techniques, or improved sleep practices, exercise complements these strategies, amplifying their effects and paving a smoother path to migraine relief.

In conclusion, embracing regular physical activity requires a commitment and patience that pays off over time. Each step taken is a stride toward not just mitigating migraines, but nurturing overall well-being. Invest in moving, breathing, and living through exercise, and you'll uncover a powerful ally in managing migraines and enhancing life quality.

Chapter 7:
Medical Treatments

Navigating the medical landscape for migraines involves understanding a plethora of available treatments, each tailored to relieve symptoms and improve quality of life. From over-the-counter remedies like ibuprofen and acetaminophen that provide accessible relief, to more potent prescription options that require thorough discussions with healthcare professionals, the spectrum of choices is vast and empowering. The key lies in collaboration with your healthcare provider to identify a plan that best suits your individual needs, balancing efficacy and potential side effects. Modern advancements also offer specialized medications targeting specific migraine mechanisms, bringing hope and relief to many. By staying informed and actively engaging with your treatment options, you can forge a path towards a life where migraines don't dictate your daily activities.

Over-the-Counter Medications

For those wrestling with the relentless grip of migraines, over-the-counter (OTC) medications can provide a lifeline—a beacon of relief amidst the storm. These widely available options serve as the first line of defense for many sufferers, offering both convenience and the promise of respite from the throbbing pain. In the landscape of migraine management, understanding the role of OTC treatments is vital. Even when these remedies might not completely eliminate symptoms, they often reduce their severity, allowing individuals to regain a sense of control.

One of the most common OTC choices is nonsteroidal anti-inflammatory drugs (NSAIDs), such as ibuprofen and aspirin. These medications work by reducing inflammation and blocking the chemical signals in the brain that trigger pain. Although primarily designed to fight inflammation, their ability to take the edge off a migraine attack has made them a staple for many. It's crucial, however, to use them correctly, as overuse can lead to medication overuse headaches—a condition that ironically exacerbates the problem you're trying to solve.

Acetaminophen, another easily accessible OTC medication, also plays a role in managing migraine symptoms. While its mechanism is somewhat different from NSAIDs, primarily targeting pain pathways in the brain, it offers a certain flexibility. It can be particularly beneficial for those who might have sensitivities or contraindications to NSAIDs. Yet, like all medications, it demands respect; excessive consumption can cause liver damage, underscoring the importance of cautious and informed use.

Combination medications, such as those pairing acetaminophen with caffeine or aspirin, provide another dimension in migraine relief strategies. Caffeine, with its vasoconstrictive properties, can help counteract the excessive dilation of blood vessels in the brain that occurs during a migraine. For some sufferers, this combination offers a more robust approach, attacking the migraine from multiple fronts. However, it's essential to be aware of caffeine's potential to contribute to rebound headaches, especially with habitual use.

The efficiency of OTC medications can vary significantly from one person to another. Some might find quick relief with a single dose, while others may need a carefully timed regime to keep an attack at bay. Factors such as the timing of the dose play a critical role; taking medication at the early onset of symptoms often proves more effective than waiting for the pain to peak. This timeliness can sometimes mean the difference between a minor inconvenience and a day rendered unbearable by migraine agony.

It's also worth discussing the importance of aligning OTC medication use with other lifestyle and medical strategies. These medications should not be seen as isolated solutions but rather as part of a broader, holistic approach to migraine management. Combining them with dietary adjustments, stress management techniques, and proper sleep routines can amplify their efficacy. In this way, they complement a more comprehensive strategy, allowing sufferers to craft a tailored path to relief.

A notable consideration is the accessibility of OTC medications. Their availability doesn't always equate to suitability, particularly when it comes to long-term use. While they can be a helpful first response, they often work best for mild to moderate migraines or as adjuncts in a longer-term treatment plan. For those with chronic migraines or more intense episodes, they may necessitate integration with prescription therapies or other medical treatments to achieve optimal results.

Migraine sufferers should approach OTC solutions with an awareness of their own bodies and health history. It's often beneficial to consult with healthcare providers—especially if there's any history of gastrointestinal issues, cardiovascular disease, or allergies that might complicate the use of certain medications. Health professionals can offer insights into safe usage, potential interactions, and alternative options if standard OTC medications prove ineffective.

Despite their potential to alleviate pain, OTC medications don't address the underlying causes of migraines. Understanding this limitation is critical, as managing triggers and identifying patterns remain key components of effective migraine management. Even as these medications provide relief, being proactive in exploring and mitigating triggers plays an equally crucial part. This dual approach—alleviating pain while seeking to understand it—empowers sufferers, offering both immediate and long-term strategies for control.

In conclusion, while OTC medications offer a practical and often necessary tool in the migraine arsenal, their use should always be informed and conscientious. Balancing their benefits with an awareness of their limitations and side effects ensures sufferers can harness their power wisely. By integrating these medications within a broader framework of supportive therapies and lifestyle changes, individuals can craft a resilient, personalized approach to managing migraines. This journey, while challenging, holds the promise of relief and empowerment, transforming obstacles into stepping stones toward improved well-being.

Prescription Options

Prescription medications can be a pivotal part of managing migraines for many sufferers. The realm of prescription options is vast and finding the right one often requires a personalized approach. With a variety of medications available, it's crucial to collaborate with your healthcare provider to tailor a treatment plan that meets your individual needs. Navigating this landscape can feel overwhelming, but understanding the potential benefits, mechanisms, and considerations of different prescriptions is an empowering step.

One major class of medications used in migraine treatment is triptans. These drugs specifically target serotonin receptors in the brain, helping to block pain pathways and providing relief from migraine episodes. Known for their efficacy in treating acute migraine attacks, triptans work best when taken as soon as migraine symptoms begin. It's essential for patients to be aware of possible side effects, which can include sensations of tingling, warmth, or pressure.

However, for many, the pros of quick relief outweigh these temporary discomforts.

Another key player in the prescription arena is the group of medications known as ergotamines. While not as commonly prescribed as triptans, ergotamines can be effective for those who haven't responded to other treatments. These medications also target serotonin receptors but work in a slightly different manner. They can be particularly beneficial for migraines that are prolonged or don't respond to more conventional triptans. Patients using ergotamines should be aware of the potential for nausea and dizziness, emphasizing the need for a personalized risk-benefit analysis with their healthcare provider.

For individuals who experience frequent migraines, preventive medications might be the answer. Beta-blockers, like propranolol, are often employed to reduce the frequency and severity of migraines. Although traditionally used for heart-related conditions, they can regulate blood flow and reduce stress responses, which may help in migraine prevention. It's important to discuss potential long-term use effects, such as fatigue and mood changes, ensuring this strategy aligns with one's overall health plan.

Anticonvulsant medications, such as topiramate and valproate, are also viable preventive options. Originally designed for epilepsy, these medications can stabilize neural activity and reduce migraine occurrence. While generally effective, they may come with a host of side effects ranging from weight changes to cognitive impacts. Continuous dialogue with a healthcare provider aids in monitoring these effects and adjusting dosage or medication type as needed.

Calcium channel blockers are another category used in migraine prevention, working by altering the way calcium travels in blood vessels, ultimately leading to fewer migraine episodes. Though not the first line of defense, they offer an alternative for those who cannot tolerate other medications. As with any medication, understanding the possible side effects, including lower blood pressure and constipation, helps set realistic expectations and vigilant monitoring.

In the realm of chronic migraine management, CGRP (Calcitonin Gene-Related Peptide) inhibitors have emerged as a groundbreaking option. These medications, such as erenumab and fremanezumab, represent a class specifically targeting migraine pathways. Administered via injection, CGRP inhibitors are designed for those with frequent migraines, offering hope for those who've had limited success with other preventatives. Patients should work closely with their healthcare team to assess the long-term implications and gauge effectiveness over time.

For some, medication tailored to coexisting conditions proves beneficial. Antidepressants, like amitriptyline, can serve a dual purpose in addressing migraines and enriching mental health. This approach highlights the intricate relationship between neurological and psychological well-being. Though effective, these medications require careful consideration of dosages and potential effects such as drowsiness and dry mouth.

Prescription options also include non-oral forms, catering to those who experience nausea and vomiting during migraines. Nasal sprays and injections provide alternatives that bypass the digestive system, ensuring faster absorption and relief. Sumatriptan, available as a nasal spray, exemplifies a solution for those who can't take pills during an attack, emphasizing the importance of flexible strategies tailored to individual experiences.

Notably, the exploration of prescription options should always be an open dialogue with your healthcare provider. Communicating honestly about any side effects, preferences, and overall responses is key to refining your treatment plan. Together, you can navigate side effects management, dosage adjustments, and select the appropriate type of medication that aligns with your lifestyle and health status.

The diversity of prescription options ensures that there's a potential solution for everyone, even if it requires some trial and error to find. Migraines, while challenging, are not insurmountable. With diligent care, support from healthcare professionals, and a proactive approach to exploring these prescriptions, sufferers can significantly manage and improve their condition. Embrace this journey with an open mind and empower yourself with knowledge, knowing there is a path forward.

Chapter 8:
Alternative Therapies

In the quest to alleviate the persistent and often debilitating symptoms of migraines, many individuals find solace in alternative therapies. Whether it's through the ancient art of acupuncture or the subtle power of herbal supplements, these approaches offer avenues to enhance well-being without solely relying on traditional medical treatments. By engaging with these therapies, one may discover unexpected benefits—like enhanced relaxation and a newfound sense of control over one's health. With growing research and anecdotal evidence supporting their potential, these therapies have become more than just a complementary option; they pave the way for holistic healing. For many, the journey through alternative therapies is not just about symptom relief but also about embracing a mindful lifestyle that cultivates balance and resilience. As you explore these therapies, you're taking an active role in your health journey, discovering tools that might just hold the key to managing your migraines more effectively. This chapter seeks to illuminate these paths, offering insights and possibilities to transform your migraine management strategy.

Acupuncture

For centuries, acupuncture has intrigued many as a distinctive therapeutic approach, an ancient practice rooted deeply in traditional Chinese medicine. But how can inserting thin needles into specific points on the body possibly alleviate the agony of migraines? It's this promising enigma that draws countless migraine sufferers to consider acupuncture as a viable alternative to conventional treatments, seeking relief where other methods have left them wanting.

The foundation of acupuncture lies in the concept of Qi (pronounced "chee")—an essential life force that flows through pathways in the body called meridians. When this flow is disrupted or blocked, it is thought to cause ailments like pain and illness. Acupuncture aims to restore the natural balance of Qi by stimulating specific points on these meridians, thus promoting healing and alleviating discomfort.

Contrary to the skepticism that accompanies many alternative therapies, acupuncture has garnered substantial scientific interest. Numerous studies suggest it might reduce the frequency and intensity of migraines and tension headaches in some individuals. The exact mechanisms behind its effectiveness are still under exploration, but theories abound, ranging from the release of endorphins to the modulation of neurotransmitter levels, providing a calming effect on the nervous system.

Those living with migraines often describe the condition as having unpredictable attacks that disrupt life unexpectedly. Acupuncture offers a sense of ritual and rhythm, a regular treatment that becomes a cornerstone in their management strategy. Whether you find yourself lying in a treatment room with soft music playing or a gentle breeze rustling outside, acupuncture allows for a moment of peace in a hectic world.

The process itself is usually well-tolerated and can even feel oddly relaxing. Practitioners select precise points on the body based on individual symptoms and overall health, inserting hair-thin needles lightly into the skin. These needles may be left in place for a few minutes to over an hour, depending on the treatment plan. Surprisingly, the sensation is often described not as painful, but as a unique tingling or warmth, evoking a mysterious dance between science and art.

Each session is an opportunity to dialogue with your body, to listen closely to its subtle cues. In this partnership between practitioner and patient, acupuncture becomes not just about physical relief, but an exercise in mindfulness, prompting patients to become more attuned to changes in their condition and their understanding of pain.

It is, however, essential to approach acupuncture with realistic expectations. While some individuals experience significant relief, others may notice changes only over time or find it less effective than hoped. Chronic migraine sufferers may opt to incorporate acupuncture as a complementary treatment, alongside other lifestyle modifications, dietary considerations, and stress management strategies. By embracing a holistic approach, they can tailor their migraine management to navigate life with as much grace and as little pain as possible.

Before starting acupuncture, it's advisable to consult with a healthcare provider to ensure that it's suitable for your specific health needs. Additionally, when selecting an acupuncturist, look for someone who is certified and has experience working with migraine sufferers, as their expertise can significantly impact your experience and results.

In closing, acupuncture stands as a beacon of hope within the realm of alternative therapies. It offers an intriguing blend of ancient wisdom and modern relevance in the quest for migraine relief. For many, it's more than just an investment in health; it's an invitation to explore new dimensions of healing, an empowering choice in one's journey to reclaim life from the clutches of migraines.

Herbal Supplements

Navigating life with migraines can be like attempting to untangle a particularly stubborn knot. What works for one person may not work for another, which is why many turn to alternative therapies, such as herbal supplements, in their quest for relief. Delving into the natural world of herbs offers promise and hope, particularly for those seeking relief beyond traditional medications that sometimes come with unwanted side effects.

A wide array of herbal supplements are touted for their potential benefits in managing migraines. Among the most popular is *Feverfew*, a small flowering plant that has become something of a staple in migraine management. Feverfew has been used for centuries in traditional medicine, especially in European countries. Research suggests that it may help in reducing both the frequency and severity of migraine attacks by inhibiting the production of certain chemicals associated with pain and inflammation.

Another cornerstone in herbal migraine management is *Butterbur*. Butterbur is a perennial plant native to Europe and parts of Asia, often found by rivers and marshes. Its appeal lies in its ability to act as a strong anti-inflammatory agent. Several studies indicate that Butterbur, when standardized to contain petasins, can effectively reduce the frequency of migraine attacks. However, it is crucial to ensure that the supplement is free of pyrrolizidine alkaloids (PAs) due to potential liver toxicity concerns.

Despite the promise these herbs offer, it's essential to approach them with caution. Just as with conventional medications, herbal supplements can interact with other treatments and may not be suitable for everyone. Consulting a healthcare provider before starting any herbal supplement is paramount, especially since the quality and potency of herbal supplements can vary significantly between brands.

Riboflavin, also known as Vitamin B2, while not an herb, often finds itself in the conversation around supplements for migraine prevention. It is believed that riboflavin helps improve mitochondrial energy efficiency, and some studies have shown that high doses may reduce the frequency of migraines. Because it's a vitamin, the risk of side effects or interactions is relatively low, making it a promising option for many sufferers.

Then there's the matter of *Magnesium*, another non-herbal supplement that's vital for a myriad of bodily functions. Its role in migraine prevention appears to be linked to its ability to influence neurotransmitter release and reduce cortical spreading depression, an event involved in migraine pathophysiology. Magnesium supplementation can be particularly beneficial for those with a deficiency, which some migraine sufferers seem to share.

Allowing ourselves to explore these natural options emphasizes our commitment to a holistic approach to health: one where knowledge, tradition, and science converge. Alongside trying these supplements, keeping track of how they affect each individual's migraine patterns can provide valuable insights over time.

It's worth remembering, though, that herbal medicine is just one piece of the puzzle. These remedies should ideally be considered part of an integrated approach, complementing other strategies such as stress management, dietary changes, and regular physical activity. This multifaceted method could potentially provide a more effective and sustainable pathway to managing migraines.

Moreover, the narrative surrounding herbal supplements isn't just about efficacy; it's about empowerment. By understanding and exploring these options, individuals gain agency over their health management processes, potentially unlocking new avenues for symptom relief.

Ultimately, the journey with herbal supplements is as much about finding balance and harmony within ourselves as it is about alleviating pain. In a world teeming with toxins and stress, plants—nature's medicine—may offer a gentle, yet powerful reprieve. Embracing the power of nature alongside medical guidance can help transform a migraine sufferer's life into one of greater peace and control, cultivating a deeper connection with themselves and the world around them.

As always, due diligence and listening to one's own body remain key. The world of herbal supplements is vast, yet nuanced, promising but needing discernment. Recognizing and respecting this balance is a vital step towards integrating these alternative therapies into a comprehensive migraine management plan. In taking this journey, sufferers are not only seeking relief but are also becoming pioneers of their own health, advocating for themselves in a world that all too often doesn't understand the invisible battle they wage.

Chapter 9:
Coping Strategies

Embracing effective coping strategies is essential for those managing the demanding world of migraines. While each sufferer's journey is unique, certain techniques can offer significant relief and empowerment. Pain management is at the forefront, where methods such as biofeedback, gentle breathing exercises, and visualization can play pivotal roles in mitigating discomfort. Emotional support, often underestimated, can be a formidable ally too. Connecting with fellow migraine sufferers through support groups or forums offers shared experiences and practical advice, while professional counseling can help navigate the emotional terrain that migraines often bring. These strategies don't just ease the physical pain; they foster a sense of control and community, reminding individuals they're not alone in this battle. Ultimately, integrating these techniques can transform the migraine experience from overwhelming to manageable, enhancing both resilience and quality of life.

Pain Management Techniques

Migraines are more than just headaches—they're a complex condition that can dramatically affect one's quality of life. While there's no one-size-fits-all solution when it comes to pain management, a variety of techniques have emerged, broadening the avenues through which sufferers can seek relief. Understanding these techniques can make a significant difference in managing both the physical and emotional aspects of migraines.

First and foremost, effective pain management often begins with an awareness of personal triggers and symptoms. Recognizing early signs of a migraine attack can enable individuals to utilize timely intervention strategies. Many find that applying a cold compress to the head, neck, or temples can help dull the pain, providing immediate soothing effects. On the other hand, some prefer warmth, so a heated pad or taking a warm bath might do the trick. The key is to experiment with both and observe what seems to work best.

With medication regimens, careful consideration and consultation with healthcare providers are crucial. Over-the-counter pain relievers like ibuprofen or aspirin may benefit some, especially when taken at the first sign of an impending headache. However, their repeated use could lead to medication overuse headaches, a paradoxical effect migraine sufferers must be wary of. Thus, exploring prescription options like triptans, which specifically target migraine pathways, might be preferable for others.

In addition to traditional medications, emerging therapies like neuromodulation devices are gaining traction. These devices offer non-invasive options for interrupting pain signals transmitted to the brain. For those wary of daily medications or looking for supplementary methods, such devices can be a game changer. They're known for being easy to use, with minimal side effects, making them a viable choice for long-term pain management.

For those looking into more structured approaches, cognitive-behavioral therapy (CBT) can be an invaluable tool. CBT helps individuals uncover negative thought patterns that could exacerbate their perception of pain. Through this therapy, sufferers learn to reframe these thoughts, thereby potentially reducing the intensity and duration of their episodes. Moreover, it equips people with coping strategies, fostering a stronger sense of control over their condition.

On a more holistic level, integrating physical therapies like physiotherapy or chiropractic treatment into one's routine can enhance pain management. These therapies focus on alleviating physical tension, improving posture, and increasing blood flow, which may reduce the frequency of migraine episodes. Many find relief in regular massage therapy, which acts as both a preventative measure and a reactive technique when used during an aura or mild attack.

Furthermore, exploring the realm of alternative medicine can open doors to unconventional yet effective methods of pain management. Acupuncture, for instance, has long been used to manage various types of pain, including migraines. By stimulating specific points on the body, acupuncture is believed to release endorphins and alter the brain's pain processing pathways. Another practice worth considering is yoga, known not only for its physical benefits but also for promoting deeper relaxation and stress relief.

An often-overlooked aspect of pain management is the role of nutrition. Certain dietary adjustments can have a profound impact on migraine reduction. Staying well-hydrated, maintaining balanced blood sugar levels, and avoiding known food triggers can support overall wellness. Some individuals find supplements like magnesium or riboflavin beneficial, though it's wise to discuss these with a healthcare provider to tailor choices to personal needs.

Equally important is building a support network, be it through family, friends, or migraine support groups. Sharing experiences and strategies with others who understand the struggle can lessen feelings of isolation and provide innovative solutions gleaned from collective wisdom. These connections serve as emotional anchors, offering encouragement and shared insights that empower individuals in their journey.

There's no doubt that managing migraine pain requires a multifaceted strategy. From medical to behavioral approaches to lifestyle changes, each technique plays a role in the overarching goal of diminishing pain and restoring a sense of normalcy. The path to effective pain management is highly individualistic—what works wonders for one might not aid another—but through diligent exploration and open-mindedness, relief is achievable. The aim is not only to reduce the frequency and severity of attacks but also to cultivate resilience and a proactive mindset in tackling migraines as part of everyday life.

Emotional Support

Living with migraines can often feel like battles fought in solitude. Due to the unpredictable nature and invisible symptoms, the struggle is largely a personal one. Yet, emotional support is vital. It can make all the difference between feeling isolated and empowered. Cultivating emotional support revolves around building a network that's empathetic, informed, and responsive to your unique experiences.

Supportive relationships are key in managing the emotional toll of chronic migraines. Friends and family, when informed and compassionate, can provide significant relief through understanding and practical help. The simple act of having someone listen, without the need to offer solutions, can be profoundly therapeutic. Conveying your experiences to those around you, however challenging it may be, creates a foundation for genuine support.

It's important to communicate your needs effectively to your support network. This can involve explaining how migraines affect you, the triggers to avoid, and how they can assist during an attack. Sometimes, this might mean asking them to help with household chores, handling loud noises, or providing a quiet space for rest. The key is to be clear and direct about what genuinely helps.

Participating in support groups, either in-person or online, can also offer solace and solidarity. Among others who truly understand the debilitating nature of migraines, you may find shared experiences, advice, and a platform to express your own journey. These groups can dispel feelings of isolation by reminding you that you're not alone in this journey.

Healthcare professionals also play a crucial role in offering emotional support. A doctor who listens and validates your symptoms, a psychologist who helps you navigate anxiety associated with migraines, or a therapist who provides coping strategies can greatly enhance your emotional well-being. Don't hesitate to reach out for professional support to better align your mental health needs with your physical condition.

At times, embracing emotional support means setting boundaries. Protecting your mental health might involve limiting interactions that lead to stress or misunderstanding. This could be as simple as excusing yourself from social gatherings that heighten your triggers or opting out of commitments that may be too taxing. Remember, it's not selfish to prioritize your health.

Cultivating a routine that encompasses self-care is equally pivotal. This routine may include activities that reduce stress and promote happiness, such as meditation, journaling, or engaging with a beloved hobby. Such practices nurture emotional resilience, allowing you to navigate the emotional highs and lows of living with migraines more effectively.

Artistic and creative outlets offer another avenue for emotional expression. Whether it's through painting, writing, or music, these activities provide a voice to the often silent battle against migraines. They allow you to articulate feelings in a way that words might sometimes fail to capture. This form of support, turning pain into creativity, fosters empowerment.

Mindfulness practices can help too. By fostering awareness and acceptance of the present moment, mindfulness exercises can alleviate the stress and anxiety that often accompany chronic migraines. This approach encourages a gentle acknowledgment of your condition, promoting peace and calm rather than frustration and anger.

The journey to integrating emotional support into your life involves patience and persistence. It's about learning how to communicate your needs, finding solace in shared understanding, and nurturing your emotional landscape with kind-hearted practices. Gradually, these efforts can transform the way you experience and manage your migraines, turning a daily struggle into a series of manageable moments.

Ultimately, the message is clear: you don't have to go through this alone. By leveraging the emotional support around you, whether it's loved ones, professional connections, or community groups, you can carve a path of resilience and strength. In the realm of chronic migraines, emotional support is not just an auxiliary component—it is an essential pillar to building a life that's not only manageable but fulfilled.

Chapter 10:
Migraine Journals

In the journey to conquer migraines, migraine journals stand out as an empowering ally, transforming your experience into actionable patterns of insight. The simple act of recording details about each migraine episode—like duration, intensity, food intake, stress levels, and sleep habits—can unveil hidden triggers and trends. By maintaining a detailed journal, you're not merely chronicling your pain, but rather crafting a personalized roadmap towards understanding and managing your migraines. It becomes an invaluable tool, helping you advocate for yourself during healthcare visits, and enables more informed discussions with your medical team. It's not just about data collection; it's about reclaiming control, illuminating the connection between daily habits and headache patterns, and guiding you towards more effective, tailored interventions.

Tracking Patterns

Embarking on the journey of understanding migraines, it's essential to recognize that these unpredictable conditions can have a more discernible rhythm and pattern than they might initially appear. The power of tracking patterns lies not only in identifying triggers but in painting a clearer picture of one's migraine landscape. This practice is transformative, offering migraine sufferers an invaluable tool that enables proactive rather than reactive behavior.

At the heart of a migraine journal is the commitment to consistent documentation. This consistency transforms scattered details into a coherent narrative, unveiling patterns that might otherwise remain hidden. When you record not just the onset of migraines but also accompanying details—like sleep quality, food intake, stress levels, and hormonal changes—you begin to see correlations that might have been overlooked. It becomes a detective story where, slowly but surely, clues are pieced together until the culprit is revealed.

Consider, for instance, the correlation between migraine occurrences and sleep disruptions. For many, maintaining a sleep journal alongside a migraine journal reveals a strong connection between restless nights and headache-filled days. Recognizing this pattern empowers individuals to prioritize sleep hygiene, perhaps leading to fewer migraine episodes. Documentation here is not just data collection; it's a strategic measure paving the way for effective interventions.

An essential aspect of this meticulous record-keeping is its potential to illuminate the subtle triggers that—while not immediately obvious—have a profound cumulative impact. For example, someone might notice that their migraines tend to spike around certain seasons, revealing environmental triggers such as pollen or temperature changes. Another person may find that their migraines follow a pattern linked to their menstrual cycle, highlighting hormonal influences.

Tracking doesn't confine itself to physical factors alone. It extends into emotional territories, shedding light on how stress and emotional upheaval can manifest physically. Perhaps there's a repeated pattern of migraines following heightened periods of anxiety or after intense emotional events. By observing these connections, it becomes easier to implement proactive stress management techniques or seek support before the physical symptoms take hold.

While digital tools and apps provide convenience and ease of tracking, many find that keeping a handwritten journal fosters a more intimate and reflective experience. Writing by hand can encourage deeper awareness and reflection, something digital entries may not always prompt. It's about finding what works best for you, ensuring the method chosen is one that encourages consistency and honesty. Whether it's a digital platform that offers reminders or a classic notebook beside your bed, the commitment to regular entry remains the cornerstone.

The patterns revealed through diligent tracking serve a dual purpose. Not only do they empower individuals to make informed lifestyle changes, but they also become a crucial resource during consultations with healthcare providers. Detailed records enhance communication, offering healthcare professionals insights that aid in tailoring treatment plans more effectively. Such information can help in deciding whether to pursue certain medications, adjust current treatments, or explore alternative therapies.

Moreover, journals extend beyond individual patterns, contributing to the broader understanding of migraines. By sharing data—either anonymously through research studies or with healthcare communities—individuals help build a more comprehensive picture of migraines, benefitting the collective knowledge pool and supporting future breakthroughs in migraine management and treatment.

It's important, during this journey of tracking and observation, to maintain a compassionate and patient approach. Perfection isn't the goal—persistence is. It's natural to encounter days where recording every detail seems overwhelming. On such days, focus on key insights; sometimes, noting just a few critical aspects can still reveal important patterns over time.

The reward of tracking extends beyond the state of physical health into mental and emotional realms as well. There is a particular reassurance in having a tangible item to refer to. It diminishes feelings of helplessness by making the intangible aspects of migraines—often felt but hard to grasp—real and actionable. This practice reinforces the notion that while migraine patterns may be complicated, they are not beyond comprehension or influence.

Each person's migraine journey is unique, and the patterns observed will not only guide individual management strategies but will also inspire personal empowerment. By honoring these insights, you may discover not just ways to alleviate pain, but also deeper connections to lifestyle elements that foster well-being. In this way, the migraine journal becomes more than a record of discomfort—it evolves into a gateway to a holistic strategy for health and wellness, one entry at a time.

Analyzing Triggers

For individuals living with migraines, identifying what prompts these debilitating episodes can be a game-changer. This journey often begins with a thorough analysis of triggers—a process that transforms vague suspicions into actionable insights. Striking patterns frequently emerge when observations are meticulously recorded, offering a clearer understanding of migraine catalysts. Recognition of these patterns is the first step toward managing and potentially reducing the frequency and intensity of attacks.

A migraine journal acts as an invaluable tool in this exploration. By logging details such as food intake, sleep patterns, stress levels, weather conditions, and more, sufferers can begin to notice correlations. Consider the way meteorologists study weather patterns to predict storms. Similarly, your journal can help forecast the likelihood of migraines by revealing which factors most commonly lead to an episode.

One cannot overlook the power of this detailed approach. When patterns are too subtle to detect through memory alone, written documentation proves indispensable. For instance, you may find that your migraines align with changes in barometric pressure or coincide with particular life stressors. Writing these details in a journal empowers you to make informed adjustments to your routine, which can lessen migraine attacks over time.

How does one start this process? Begin with commitment and consistency. Make it a daily ritual to jot down key information. While it may initially feel like an additional chore, the benefits can be transformative. In the short term, the data may appear chaotic, but over weeks or months, patterns become discernible. Perhaps there's a delayed reaction to a specific food, or a reliable response during particular phases of the menstrual cycle.

It's important to include a comprehensive range of potential triggers in your analysis. Environmental factors like bright lights or loud noises, emotional stressors, dietary choices, and hormonal changes should all be considered. The role technology can play should not be underestimated either; various apps can help streamline this process, making logging quicker and analyses more sophisticated.

Moreover, sharing your findings with healthcare providers can be immensely beneficial. They can offer professional insights, assisting you in identifying triggers that may not be apparent at first glance. This collaborative approach harnesses your experiential knowledge and their medical expertise, ultimately refining your overall migraine management plan.

Yet, one must approach this venture with an open mind and patience. Not every identified factor will cause migraines every time, as triggers can be fickle and context-dependent. The interplay between multiple triggers sometimes causes an attack, rather than one single trigger acting in isolation. This complexity requires a persistent, detailed, and sometimes experimental approach to truly understand.

Your analytical journey is also paved with personal anecdotes and stories. By sharing experiences with support groups, either online or in person, you gain both motivation and potentially, new insights. Collective wisdom amplifies individual understanding, reinforcing awareness that while migraines are uniquely personal, there's strength in community learning and support.

Accumulating data over time allows for deeper insights into secondary triggers—those that might not initiate a migraine but exacerbate one. Identifying such factors can help reduce the severity of attacks. For instance, a minor headache may intensify into a full-blown migraine under the influence of additional triggers like caffeine or lack of sleep.

This deep dive into self-awareness can also prompt lifestyle changes. Imagine discovering that skipped meals are a trigger; this insight nudges toward more regular eating habits. In such ways, analyzing triggers fosters proactive behavior, leading to healthier overall routines and improved quality of life.

As you venture into analyzing triggers, maintain a balance between focus and flexibility. Recognizing unique patterns within your experience encourages adaptability. Remember that as life changes, so can triggers, emphasizing the need for continuous observation and adaptation.

Migraines make daily life challenging, but a diligent approach to analyzing triggers can turn understanding them from an elusive task into an achievable goal. Armed with knowledge, you hold the key to reducing your migraine burden significantly, thereby enriching your journey toward a more manageable existence.

Chapter 11:
Working with Healthcare Teams

Partnering effectively with healthcare teams can be a game changer in the journey of managing migraines. It's not just about finding a doctor who knows about migraines; it's about establishing a robust support network that genuinely understands your unique challenges. Communication is key, and clear, open dialogue with your healthcare providers can lead to more personalized treatment plans that align with your lifestyle and needs. Engage actively in discussions about your symptoms, treatments you've tried, and any side effects you're experiencing. This transparency helps your healthcare team tailor interventions that can significantly reduce the frequency and intensity of your migraines. Remember, you're not alone in this journey—embrace your role in this partnership to empower yourself and improve your quality of life. Together with your healthcare team, you can navigate through this condition with greater confidence and resilience.

Building a Support Network

In the complex journey of managing migraines, building a robust support network is nothing short of essential. Navigating the healthcare landscape requires not only the expertise of medical professionals but the genuine understanding and assistance of people who care about you. Establishing this network goes beyond mere convenience; it's about creating a system of emotional and practical support that can significantly enhance your quality of life.

The foundation of any effective support network for migraine sufferers starts with open communication. Sharing your experiences, frustrations, and victories with those around you can foster understanding and empathy. Begin with family and close friends, inviting them into your journey. Educate them about migraines in a way that resonates, perhaps by comparing the experience to something relatable in their lives. Awareness and empathy go hand in hand, and when people around you grasp the intricacies of migraines, they can provide the support that's truly needed.

Your healthcare team plays an indispensable role in your support network. This includes not just your primary care physician, but also specialists like neurologists, dietitians, and mental health counselors. Each member of this team offers expertise tailored to different aspects of migraine management. It's crucial to feel empowered to ask questions and express concerns to these professionals, ensuring that your treatment plan is continuously aligned with your personal needs and goals.

Community groups and support networks offer another layer of connection. Whether meeting in person or engaging in online forums, connecting with fellow migraine sufferers can be both healing and validating. These communities provide a space where you can share experiences, swap coping strategies, and even just vent. Knowing that others share your struggles can reduce feelings of isolation, reinforcing that you are not alone in this journey.

Meanwhile, professional organizations devoted to migraine research and support can be invaluable resources. They often host seminars, workshops, and webinars that provide the latest information on migraine management. Engaging with such organizations keeps you informed about new treatments and research developments, equipping you with knowledge that could be a game-changer in managing your condition.

The workplace is another sphere where your support network can be impactful. While navigating work with migraines can be challenging, having understanding colleagues and an inclusive employer makes a significant difference. Don't hesitate to communicate your needs and discuss accommodations that could help you maintain productivity without compromising your health. Whether it's modifying your workspace or adjusting work hours, even small changes can have a profound impact on your well-being.

External relationships like friendships and social connections must also be nurtured thoughtfully. Be open with your friends about your condition and the limitations it sometimes imposes. Suggest alternatives if certain activities are likely to trigger your migraines. This proactive approach not only helps in maintaining social bonds but also sets realistic expectations, reducing stress for all involved.

Your support network also serves as a safety net. In times of severe migraines, knowing you have people to count on can be a comfort all its own. It's important to designate a few key people who can step in during emergencies, helping with tasks that may be difficult or impossible when you're in the throes of a migraine attack. This could include picking up prescriptions, driving you to appointments, or just being present to help you manage through the pain.

It's equally important to ensure that your support network is reciprocal and dynamic. This means not only leaning on others in times of need but also maintaining your connections by returning support whenever you're able. This balance ensures that your relationships remain healthy and sustainable, fostering trust and mutual respect.

Over time, your support network may change and adapt, much like your treatment plan. People might come and go, healthcare professionals might change, and you may discover new resources that better fit your evolving needs. Embrace this evolution, being open to new relationships and perspectives that could enrich your journey.

As you build and refine your support network, remember that the key is communication, openness, and willingness to both give and receive support. With a strong network, you are not just building connections; you are creating a resilient framework that bolsters your ability to manage migraines effectively.

The road to managing migraines is undeniably challenging, but with the right support system by your side, it becomes a shared journey rather than a solitary path. In these partnerships, you find strength, cultivate hope, and ultimately empower yourself to take control of your health and your life.

Effective Communication

In the realm of managing migraines, particularly when working with a healthcare team, effective communication is the cornerstone of successful treatment and support. It's not just about conveying symptoms; it's about ensuring that your medical needs and personal experiences with migraines are fully understood. This mutual understanding enables healthcare professionals to develop a treatment plan that is tailored, comprehensive, and effective.

Many migraine sufferers find that articulating the specifics of their condition can be daunting. The episodic nature of migraines often makes it challenging to convey the variability and intensity of symptoms. Therefore, it's essential to prepare for conversations with healthcare providers by keeping a detailed migraine journal. This journal should track not only the frequency and severity of your migraines but also potential triggers, dietary influences, and emotional states associated with each episode. Such detailed records can provide valuable insights, turning subjective experiences into objective information that doctors can use to refine and adjust treatment strategies.

Creating a dialogue rather than a monologue is vital in conversations with healthcare teams. This involves asking questions about proposed treatments, expressing concerns if a certain approach seems unsuitable, and being open about what has or hasn't worked in the past. It's okay to challenge ideas or ask for alternatives if something doesn't resonate with you. Healthcare providers are there to guide you, but your input about your own experience is invaluable.

Anxiety or fatigue from discussing painful episodes can sometimes render these interactions difficult. Preparation is crucial. Practice explaining your situation clearly and concisely. Consider writing down points you want to discuss. When you're well-prepared, it's easier to focus on the conversation and advocate for your health needs effectively.

Effective communication also includes listening—really listening. Understand the advice, educate yourself on your condition and treatment options, and don't hesitate to ask for clarification if medical jargon becomes overwhelming. Remember, a good healthcare provider will appreciate a patient who seeks comprehension rather than compliance.

Building rapport with your healthcare team can go a long way. Consistent, respectful communication fosters trust, which can be crucial when decisions about more aggressive treatments or lifestyle changes are discussed. In times of crisis, a strong patient-provider relationship can be the difference between a manageable situation and a stressful experience.

Also, consider involving family members or friends in some of your appointments. They can provide support, help remember details, and offer additional perspectives that might be beneficial to your healthcare provider. Their involvement may also help them understand what you're going through, which can be particularly comforting during migraine episodes.

Of course, not every interaction with the healthcare system will be smooth. Miscommunication might happen, or you might encounter a professional who doesn't share your views. In these cases, staying calm and reiterating your points is key. Document any discrepancies for future reference, and don't hesitate to seek a second opinion if you feel your concerns aren't being addressed adequately.

Effective communication is not limited to face-to-face appointments. With advances in technology, many healthcare providers offer telemedicine consultations, which can be particularly beneficial if you are experiencing a migraine. Setting up a comfortable environment for these virtual appointments can help ensure you remain focused and effective in communicating your needs.

Furthermore, some migraine-specific apps offer ways to track symptoms and medication use, which can be shared directly with your healthcare team. These digital tools can enhance communication by providing real-time data that healthcare providers can use to adjust treatment plans more effectively.

Beyond the practicalities, maintaining hope and a positive outlook is crucial. Building a transparent and trusting relationship with healthcare professionals involved in your care gives you a sense of agency, an essential component in managing a chronic condition like migraines. You're part of a team working towards the same goal: reducing the frequency and severity of your migraines to improve your quality of life.

In summary, effective communication is more than just exchanging words. It's an ongoing process of collaboration, understanding, and mutual respect between you and your healthcare team. With clear and open communication, you empower yourself as an active participant in your healthcare journey, ultimately paving the way for more effective management of your migraines.

Chapter 12:
Navigating Social Situations

Migraines aren't just about intense headaches; they impact social interactions and relationships, too. When you're at a lively gathering, the last thing you want is a migraine to darken your enjoyment. It's important to communicate openly with those around you. Explain your condition honestly and discuss the triggers that might lurk in social environments, like loud music or harsh lighting. This awareness helps others understand the invisible challenges you face. Prioritize self-care; it's okay to leave early or skip an event if you need to. You're training those around you to respect your limits, setting an example for self-advocacy. Remember, maintaining a supportive social circle can be a pivotal anchor in managing your migraines, making the burden feel a little lighter.

Explaining Migraines to Others

It's difficult to convey the complex reality of living with migraines to those who haven't experienced them, yet it's crucial for easing social interactions and gaining the understanding you need. Many people mistakenly equate migraines with mere headaches or temporary discomfort, and this misunderstanding often leads to a lack of empathy and support. Educating others about the true nature of migraines starts with emphasizing their debilitating impact. Migraines can be paralyzing, disrupting daily life with intense headaches, visual disturbances, nausea, and extreme sensitivity to light and sound, among other symptoms.

Begin with clear communication. Use straightforward language to describe what a migraine feels like for you. Words like "throbbing," "pulsating," or "piercing" can help illustrate the severity and unpredictability of migraine pain. Compare it to recognizable experiences if that helps, like the kind of disorientation someone might feel after hours of staring at a computer screen without breaks. Explaining the variability of migraine triggers and symptoms can also be enlightening for those unfamiliar with this condition. Pointing out that what works one day might not work the next conveys the challenge of managing such an unpredictable condition.

Possibly the greatest communication hurdle is making others see that you're not exaggerating or using migraines as an excuse. Encourage empathy by emphasizing the ripple effects of a migraine attack. For example, missing out on family occasions, having to leave work early, or needing solitude can create feelings of isolation and guilt. Highlighting these emotional components helps convey that migraines are more than just a physical ailment.

Personal anecdotes can be powerful. Share a story of a time when a migraine interrupted something important. This personal touch can engage the listener, making the issue feel more real and less abstract. Personal stories emphasize the unpredictability and uncontrollability of migraine attacks. Whether it was having to leave a concert, missing a birthday party, or needing to cancel plans with friends, these stories often resonate on a human level and evoke understanding.

Finding the appropriate moment to discuss your migraines matters. If a migraine is triggered at a social gathering, for instance, explaining what's happening can be far more effective when emotions and pain levels are manageable. Clear, calm communication is generally more constructive than trying to explain while overwhelmed.

It also helps to provide factual information. Share that migraines affect millions and are recognized as one of the most debilitating illnesses globally, according to the World Health Organization. People often respond well to medical facts, as they validate your condition and stress its seriousness. Knowledge from a credible source can make others take your condition more seriously.

Visual aids can be particularly useful. Consider showing diagrams of the brain during an attack or sharing an article that outlines migraine phases. Often, seeing something in print or visuals helps solidify an understanding that words alone might not achieve.

Beyond direct communication, it can be beneficial to enlist allies who understand your situation, like family members or close friends who can vouch for your experience. They can support you by explaining your situation to others, helping lift that burden from you. This way, you're also building a more informed community around you, which is invaluable.

Remember to express gratitude when someone shows understanding or goes out of their way to accommodate your needs. Positive reinforcement encourages continued support and empathy, showing them that their efforts make a tangible difference in your life.

Since migraines can alter plans at a moment's notice, establishing open channels of communication with those you socialize with regularly is crucial. Let them know it's nothing personal when you have to withdraw from activities. Honest communication helps build trust and minimizes any misconceptions that might arise over time.

In some scenarios, using written communication can be advantageous, especially at work or in formal settings where verbal explanation isn't feasible. An email or note can succinctly lay out your situation, making it easier for people to process and refer back to.

Ultimately, explaining migraines to others is about advocating for yourself. Building a bridge to understanding can foster increased tolerance and empathy, making your social interactions smoother and less stressful. With time and persistence, those who matter will learn to appreciate the realities of your condition, transforming confusion into compassion and skepticism into support.

Social Settings and Triggers

Migraines, with their unpredictable nature, can transform a bustling social event into a personal ordeal. Imagine being at a family wedding, surrounded by the laughter of loved ones and the clinking of champagne glasses, only to feel the sudden, throbbing onset of a migraine. What begins as a celebration can quickly spiral into an overwhelming sensory attack. Recognizing how social settings can trigger migraines is crucial for those who wish to participate in life's joyful moments while managing their symptoms effectively.

Social gatherings often come with a myriad of potential migraine triggers. Bright lights, loud music, and crowds can easily overstimulate the brain, setting the stage for an attack. For many, it's not just one factor—it's the combination of several that tips the scales. Consider a night out with friends. The dim but flashing club lights, the reverberating bass, and the swirl of dancing figures—all potent enough alone—become a perfect storm when combined. It's no surprise that some migraine sufferers might feel hesitant to even consider such outings.

Alcohol, another staple of many social settings, deserves special mention. While one drink might relax the mind, for some, it's a double-edged sword. Alcohol, especially red wine and beer, is a well-documented migraine trigger, sometimes causing or intensifying an episode within hours. While the social pressures to partake are intense, understanding and asserting your boundaries can make all the difference.

On the flip side, the lack of control in many social situations can escalate stress levels, which is another common trigger. When attending events organized by others, you might feel confined by their schedules and preferences. What if the music is too loud, or the meal triggers a migraine due to an allergy or sensitivity? The concern over these unknowns can inadvertently lead to the very condition you're hoping to avoid.

Effective communication becomes your best tool in managing these situations. Informing close friends or family about your condition can foster an environment of understanding. It's beneficial to have at least one person aware of your early warning signs and strategies to mitigate them. Simple arrangements, like securing a quiet space for retreat or ensuring non-alcoholic options are available, can offer a semblance of control.

When preparing to attend a social event, planning can serve as a valuable ally. Consider timeframes and environments when you're less likely to experience a migraine. If evenings are typically challenging, perhaps suggest afternoon gatherings. Additionally, if you know that skipping meals or fluctuating blood sugar levels trigger your symptoms, prepare by eating a balanced snack before attending the event.

Despite all precautions, sometimes migraines will still break through, stubbornly ignoring our best-laid plans. In these moments, it's essential to carry a migraine toolkit—a small pouch containing essentials like prescribed medications, a comfortable eye mask, earplugs, or noise-canceling headphones. Having these items on hand isn't an admission of defeat; rather, it's a proactive approach to maintaining agency over your well-being.

Building resilience in social settings is as much about mindset as it is about actions. Redefining success can mitigate the guilt associated with leaving early or canceling plans. Rather than viewing these instances as failures, consider them victories in self-care. Engaging with support groups can also be a transformative experience. Sharing strategies and stories, either in person or online, offers both reassurance and practical insights from those who understand the challenges firsthand.

It's also worth exploring environments that are naturally accommodating for migraine sufferers. Outdoor gatherings, like picnics or walks in a park, provide a perfect backdrop with natural light and expansive spacing. If indoors, selecting venues with controlled lighting and sound settings can be a game-changer.

Finally, it's crucial to foster open dialogue within your social circle. Encourage conversations about migraines, explaining the complexities and individual nature of triggers. Sharing personal experiences not only raises awareness but also cultivates empathy. It allows friends and family to appreciate that what might seem like a minor inconvenience to them can be genuinely debilitating for you.

Your journey with migraines will have its ups and downs, but with adaptive strategies and mindful preparations, social settings don't have to be overwhelming. By weaving together meticulous planning, communication, and self-awareness, you can reclaim the joy of these experiences, armed not just as a participant, but as an advocate for your own comfort and health. Every event mastered, every interaction navigated with ease, isn't just a step forward in managing migraines— it's a celebration of resilience and self-empowerment.

Chapter 13:
Migraines in the Workplace

Finding a way to manage migraines in the workplace can be challenging, yet it's essential for maintaining both productivity and well-being. Start by creating a migraine-friendly environment; subtle adjustments like tweaking lighting, reducing noise levels, and establishing a designated quiet area can make a substantial impact. It's crucial to communicate with your employer about your needs, as many are willing to provide reasonable accommodations such as flexible hours or remote work options. Don't hesitate to incorporate brief breaks and relaxation techniques into your day—they can alleviate stress and ward off impending migraine attacks. Fellow colleagues may not fully understand your struggle, so sharing insightful information about migraines can foster empathy and support. By effectively managing symptoms and leveraging employer support, you can craft a work atmosphere that doesn't compromise your health or your professional obligations.

Managing Symptoms at Work

For many people with migraines, work isn't just a source of income— it's a place where ambitions thrive and identities take shape. But when migraine symptoms hit amidst deadlines and meetings, the challenge can seem daunting. Managing these symptoms at work demands not just medical intervention but strategic adjustments to your physical and mental environment.

First, it's crucial to identify what workplace factors might trigger or exacerbate your migraines. Bright or flickering lights, loud noises, and even strong odors can be potent triggers. If your work environment includes any of these elements, consider requesting adjustments. For example, you might benefit from a desk lamp with adjustable brightness instead of relying on fluorescent lighting. Many employers are becoming increasingly aware of health considerations and might be willing to accommodate.

Effective communication remains at the heart of managing migraines in the workplace. It's not always easy to explain an invisible condition that varies in intensity and duration. However, having an honest conversation with your supervisor can lay the groundwork for necessary accommodations. Whether you require more flexible hours, the option to work from home, or simply a quiet place to recuperate during an attack, clear communication is key. Provide them with concrete examples of how these adjustments could help you maintain productivity despite migraines.

Think about creating a migraine-friendly workstation. Keeping essential tools at hand can reduce the stress of unplanned migraine attacks. Consider noise-canceling headphones if your workspace is particularly noisy, or a small fan if you're sensitive to temperature changes. Additionally, maintaining posture is crucial; ergonomic furniture or accessories like a supportive chair or a standing desk can make all the difference.

Proactive management strategies can also help prevent migraine pain from escalating during working hours. Develop a routine that includes scheduled breaks, which can help with eye strain and stress reduction. Utilizing techniques like deep-breathing exercises or quick meditation sessions can significantly reduce stress, one of the most common migraine triggers, helping you reset and recharge.

Let's not overlook the importance of hydration and nutrition. Dehydration and low blood sugar levels can be precursors to a migraine attack. Keeping a water bottle at your desk can serve as a regular reminder to hydrate. Similarly, having a stash of healthy snacks, such as nuts or fruits, can help maintain your energy levels without the risk of triggering migraines due to hunger-related stress.

Sometimes, despite the best preventive efforts, a migraine attack might occur. Having a contingency plan can help you manage these episodes with a little more ease. If you have access to a medical room or a quiet space within your workplace, using this area for a short, restorative break could be invaluable. Techniques such as lying down in a dark, quiet room (if possible) or practicing relaxation exercises may reduce the severity of the attack.

Technology can offer additional support. Utilizing apps that track your symptoms and alert you to patterns or triggers can provide valuable data. Sharing this information with your healthcare provider can lead to more personalized treatment plans. When equipped with a better understanding of your migraines, you can approach your employer with more precise requests for workplace adjustments.

It's crucial to involve your healthcare team when considering the impacts of migraines on your work life. They can provide insights and tailor treatments that accommodate your conditions within the work environment. Often, healthcare professionals can add weight to your discussions with your employer, offering written advice or recommendations that explain the seriousness of your condition.

Remember, managing migraines at work doesn't mean you have to compromise your professional growth. In fact, finding ways to effectively manage symptoms can lead to increased resilience and problem-solving skills, enhancing your career journey. You're not alone in this battle, and many people have found meaningful ways to incorporate their migraine management into their work life, ultimately improving not just their pain but their well-being too.

In short, while migraines can pose unique challenges in the workplace, there are numerous strategies that can be employed to better manage these symptoms. By understanding your triggers, communicating effectively, and developing a supportive work environment, you can continue to thrive professionally while maintaining control over your health. Above all, remember that seeking support, both medical and professional, is not a sign of weakness but a commendable step in empowering yourself against the disorder.

Employer Support and Accommodations

For many migraine sufferers, the workplace is both a source of purpose and a potential minefield of triggers. Recognizing these challenges, it's crucial to find a balance between career aspirations and health needs. Employers play a vital role in this balance, and understanding how they can offer support is key to creating a healthier work environment for everyone—even those without migraines.

Employers can begin by fostering a culture of empathy and understanding. Encouraging open conversations about migraines and other invisible illnesses helps to destigmatize these conditions. Knowledge is power, and when colleagues and supervisors know more about migraines, they're better positioned to offer meaningful support. Workshops or seminars led by healthcare professionals, either in person or virtually, can be effective. These sessions could cover the basics of what migraines are, what they are not, and how to recognize and respond to the needs of those affected.

Beyond education, practical accommodations can significantly improve a migraine sufferer's work life. Flexible working hours are a crucial step. Many find that migraines can be unpredictable, flaring up with little warning. Being able to adjust one's schedule allows the individual to work when symptoms are minimal and rest when necessary. Remote work options, which have become more prevalent, also offer a sanctuary from the potential sensory overload of a busy office environment.

Creating a migraine-friendly workspace is another supportive measure. Employers can provide dimmable lighting or reduce fluorescent light exposure when possible. Noise-canceling features in open office plans or offering quiet rooms for breaks can also mitigate one of the most common migraine triggers: noise. Additionally, ensuring adequate ventilation and maintaining a scent-free environment can further help prevent unnecessary headaches.

It's important to note that these accommodations not only enhance productivity but also boost employee morale. Workers who feel supported are generally more engaged and loyal. Implementing simple adjustments can lead to a more inclusive and efficient workplace culture that benefits everyone, not just those suffering from migraines.

Accommodations should also account for the need for occasional breaks and rest periods. A policy that allows for short, frequent breaks can help employees manage their energy levels throughout the day and reduce the likelihood of a migraine attack. Workplaces could incorporate rest areas that offer a quiet, comfortable space for rejuvenation. Encouraging regular check-ins with employees ensures that the support offered remains effective and evolves with the individual's needs.

Effective communication is the backbone of successful accommodation. Employers should encourage an open-door policy where employees feel safe discussing their health needs without fear of judgment or retribution. Confidentiality is crucial in these conversations, as it builds trust and encourages honesty. Employees should be proactive, too, clearly communicating their needs and suggesting solutions that have worked for them in the past.

Moreover, collaboration between HR departments and occupational health advisors can create customized support plans. These tailored strategies should recognize that migraines vary greatly from person to person, both in frequency and intensity. Flexibility in these plans ensures that they remain relevant and beneficial over time.

Training managers to recognize the signs of a migraine in an employee can also be beneficial. It's often about spotting subtle cues and understanding when a colleague needs a moment to step away. A sensitive approach can make all the difference in managing the impact of migraines on work life.

Incorporating technology solutions can also enhance support. Specialized apps for migraine management can be offered to employees, allowing them to log symptoms, track patterns, and even share reports with supervisors if they choose. Wearable devices that monitor stress levels, posture, and even light exposure can inform better workplace practices.

Additionally, workplace wellness programs can be tailored to include workshops on stress management, ergonomics, and healthy lifestyle practices that have been shown to reduce migraine frequency. Providing resources and access to therapies like yoga or meditation can encourage a proactive approach to health management among employees.

Implementing these strategies doesn't only benefit those with migraines—it can improve the overall workplace environment. A healthier, more understanding workplace contributes to better employee retention, reduced absenteeism, and improved team morale. The investment in accommodations and support systems highlights a commitment to employee well-being, reflecting positively on the organization's values.

Ultimately, the goal is to create an environment where every employee, migraine sufferer or not, can thrive. Achieving this means acknowledging the complexities of migraines and building a workplace that prioritizes health and compassion. When employers and employees collaborate effectively, the result is a more harmonious and productive workspace.

Chapter 14:
Travel Tips for Migraine Sufferers

Traveling with migraines doesn't have to be daunting; with a bit of foresight and the right strategies, you can journey with ease and confidence. Start by creating a personalized migraine travel kit filled with essentials like medications, hydration solutions, and soothing aids like eye masks or lavender packets. Don't forget to plan your rest stops if you're driving or choose seats with reduced motion exposure when flying, such as over the wings. It's crucial to maintain a balanced diet and stay hydrated, as neglecting these can quickly turn a getaway into a headache. Communicate your needs politely with travel companions and staff to find supportive allies who understand your situation. Above all, stay flexible and listen to your body – it's okay to take time to recuperate if needed. Embracing these tips, you can manage migraines on the move and make your travels as enjoyable as your destination.

Planning Ahead

Traveling can be a daunting task for migraine sufferers, as the unpredictability of migraines doesn't respect the excitement of a journey. However, planning ahead offers an effective strategy for managing migraines while on the go. By anticipating potential challenges and preparing for a myriad of scenarios, you can transform your travel experience from burdensome to enjoyable. Understanding the importance of comprehensive planning is crucial and can significantly reduce stress and enhance your travel quality.

The first step in planning your trip should be to conduct thorough research on your destination. This includes understanding the weather, accessibility to healthcare facilities, and access to quiet spaces where you can retreat if a migraine strikes. Knowing the climate is particularly important as weather patterns could influence your migraine triggers. Furthermore, close proximity to medical facilities is comforting, offering quick access to professional help if necessary. Similarly, identifying low-stimulation environments such as parks or gardens, libraries, or quiet cafes allows you to have a go-to place where you can find respite during your trip.

Creating a migraine travel kit is another practical step. This kit should be meticulously packed with essentials that help manage symptoms or triggers. Items could include your medications, a reusable water bottle, an eye mask, earplugs, and perhaps even a cooling gel pack. Having such a kit on hand enables swift self-care which can be crucial in nipping an attack in the bud. Don't forget to pack in multiples of your prescription medications to ensure you won't run out.

Equally vital is setting a flexible itinerary. While it's tempting to want to see and do everything, allowing room for rest and relaxation is invaluable. Building downtime into your schedule ensures you don't overexert yourself. Consider activities that align with your usual routines. If you're used to taking an afternoon nap at home, or if meditation is part of your ritual, find a way to incorporate these into your travel plans. Flights, long drives, or train rides can offer a great opportunity for rest if you prepare properly—think neck pillows, noise-canceling headphones, or soothing music to help you relax.

Travel involves a change in daily routines, and consequently, it can disrupt your sleep patterns. Given the established link between sleep and migraine onset, prioritize maintaining a consistent sleep schedule despite time zone changes. If you're traveling across time zones, gradually adjust your sleeping and eating habits a few days in advance. New environments and beds can also affect sleep quality, so consider bringing a travel-sized pillow or blanket that might provide comfort. Technology can assist here; sleep apps or white noise apps could help you ease into sleep, no matter where you are.

For those with food-related triggers, taking the time to learn about local cuisine and available dining options can be lifesaving. Research restaurants, local supermarkets, and food delivery options that offer dishes compatible with your dietary needs. If unsure, don't hesitate to communicate your requirements to the serving staff, or even employ translation apps to express your needs clearly in a different language. Snacks that are safe from your triggers, packed from home, can be lifesavers during long transits or upon reaching your destination when local options haven't been confirmed.

Being aware of your modes of transport is another crucial element of planning ahead. Different modes come with different triggers—whether it's the altitude of a plane, the motion of a boat, or the tight space in a car. Understanding personal susceptibilities can guide the choice of the best transport medium suitable for you. For air travel, booking seats that offer more leg room or are near the front to minimize motion discomfort could be beneficial. Also, checking the airline for their policies on medicines and medical devices in carry-on allowance helps avoid unnecessary stress at airport security.

Additionally, an essential, albeit often overlooked part of planning, is crafting a communication plan. Let the people you're traveling with know about your condition and how they can assist if a migraine occurs. Inform them about the specific triggers to avoid and the symptoms of an impending attack. Such communication fosters understanding and reduces potential embarrassment, providing you peace of mind. Provide them with a basic migraine response kit or list of instructions so they can be of assistance.

Furthermore, acquiring travel insurance that covers health issues, including migraines, adds a layer of security. Review policies carefully to ensure that migraines are indeed covered. This step could alleviate financial worry associated with unexpected medical consultations or interventions while you are away from home.

Lastly, mental preparation is just as crucial as logistical planning. Recognize that despite all preparation, you might still experience a migraine. Mentally accepting this possibility reduces anxiety, allowing you to enjoy the moments in between attacks more thoroughly. Mindfulness techniques can help in maintaining an optimistic outlook. As much as your physical comfort matters, nurturing positive mental resilience can provide as much relief on your travel journey.

By planning ahead effectively, traveling doesn't have to be prohibitive for migraine sufferers. Instead, it opens a world replete with adventures and new experiences, simultaneously mindful of your health needs. As you embark on your journeys, may this proactive approach to migraine management empower you to explore with confidence and assurance.

Managing Symptoms on the Go

Travel can be both exhilarating and daunting, especially for migraine sufferers. Juggling itineraries, time zones, and unfamiliar environments can easily trigger an episode. Yet, by being proactive, you can keep migraines from overshadowing your adventures. Here's how you can empower yourself to manage your symptoms effectively while on the move.

Start with a solid plan. Preparation isn't just about packing a suitcase; it's about foreseeing the potential triggers of travel. Create a checklist well ahead of your trip. This should include essential medications, sunglasses to protect against harsh lighting, and noise-canceling headphones to block sudden sounds. While it may seem excessive, having a strategy in place can be the difference between an enjoyable journey and one marked by discomfort.

Hydration is another cornerstone of managing migraines while traveling. Air travel, in particular, can be dehydrating due to dry cabin air. Aim to drink plenty of water before, during, and after your flight. Carry a reusable water bottle, filling it up whenever you have the opportunity. Dehydration is a common trigger for migraines, and staying adequately hydrated can prevent or lessen the severity of an attack.

Your travel snacks deserve attention too. While it might be tempting to indulge in airport fare or local delicacies upon arrival, be mindful of foods that could trigger your migraines. Opt for simple, familiar snacks like nuts, fruits, or whole grains. Avoid known culprits in your diet, such as chocolate, cheese, or alcohol. It's all about keeping surprises to a minimum and ensuring a stable internal environment.

Regular eating and sleeping schedules might prove challenging when on the go, but maintaining a routine can help manage migraines. Jet lag and sleepless nights can be harsh, yet they are manageable with a few tricks. Consider adjusting your watch to the destination's time zone as soon as you board the plane. Trying to eat, sleep, and wake according to your destination's time zone can help your body transition more smoothly.

In-flight comfort is vital, so consider investing in travel essentials that make a difference. A supportive neck pillow, a lightweight blanket, or an eye mask can enhance your comfort. However, don't ignore the small but crucial details like maintaining an upright posture or stretching your legs at regular intervals. Movement keeps your circulation going and minimizes tension that might lead to headaches.

Navigating through bustling airports or train stations can be overstimulating. Their bright lights, loud announcements, and throngs of people can stress an already sensitive system. Minimize exposure by wearing polarized sunglasses and using earplugs. Additionally, seek out quiet areas where you can take a breather if needed. Most transport hubs offer zones designated for peace-seeking travelers.

Even the best-laid plans can falter, so remain flexible. Accept that schedules might change and obstacles may arise. Carry a small kit that holds your go-to remedies, be that medication, aromatic oils, or a cold compress. Sometimes, retreating to a quiet, dark room, even for a few minutes, can make all the difference in warding off a full-blown migraine.

While it's natural to feel trepidation when faced with such unpredictability, remember that technology can be a helpful ally. Apps that track time zones, offer guided meditations, or provide relaxation music can ease your transition and mitigate stress. Having such digital companions can ensure your mental relaxation aligns with the physical strategies you've employed.

Social encounters and obligations often accompany travel. Be upfront with those you're with about your needs. Communicate openly about your condition and the potential necessity for breaks or specific accommodations. Most friends and colleagues will appreciate your candor and be more understanding if you plainly outline what helps or hinders your wellness.

Lastly, reflect on your journey. Consider what worked well and what didn't. Documenting this in a travel journal could illuminate patterns and preferences that could inform future trips. This practice not only aids in organizing your thoughts but serves as a valuable reference. It's about learning from each experience, adjusting strategies, and becoming more adept at managing symptoms on the go.

Travel should expand your world and offer joy, not anxiety. With mindfulness, good preparation, and adaptability, you can embrace the adventure ahead. Mastering symptom management on the road empowers you to explore without fear, nurturing a sense of confidence as you encounter the vista that awaits.

Chapter 15:
Sleep and Migraines

Understanding the intricate dance between sleep and migraines can be the key that unlocks a more peaceful existence for many sufferers. Proper sleep hygiene isn't just a wellness catchphrase here—it's a cornerstone of effective migraine management. Without adequate and restful sleep, the brain remains in a heightened state of alertness, often triggering those dreaded migraines. Creating an environment favorable to slumber involves dimming lights, reducing noise, and ensuring comfort. This isn't a luxury but an obligation to oneself. The art lies in establishing a consistent routine, as even small deviations can ripple into big consequences. Think of it as a tapestry, where each thread of your nightly ritual weaves together resilience against attacks. Embrace the night as an ally in your journey to reclaim life's vibrancy from the grip of migraines.

Importance of Sleep Hygiene

Sleep, often overlooked, plays a vital role in managing migraines. For anyone dealing with migraines, establishing a consistent sleep routine could be as crucial as their diet or medication regimen. It's fascinating how something as regular as sleep can impact our health journey. Researchers have long noted that irregular or poor sleep patterns can exacerbate migraine frequency and intensity. Ensuring that sleep contributes positively rather than negatively is where sleep hygiene becomes indispensable.

When we talk about sleep hygiene, we're referring to habits and practices conducive to sleeping well on a consistent basis. For individuals battling migraines, prioritizing sleep hygiene isn't just about increasing the quantity of sleep; it's about enhancing its quality. It's an opportunity to create a restful environment and implement practices that make restful nights more attainable. For those living with chronic headaches, reducing migraine occurrences can greatly improve daily living, making sleep a powerful tool in their arsenal.

Why does sleep hold so much power? It turns out that sleep impacts the brain's processing networks, which are intricately tied to migraine pathways. During restful sleep, the body undergoes processes that can help mitigate these pathways, reducing the potential for migraine triggers. This is why missing out on sleep or experiencing disrupted sleep can lead to an immediate rise in migraine attacks for many sufferers. Simply put, sleep acts as a reset button for the brain.

Establishing a strong sleep-wake cycle is at the heart of sleep hygiene. This includes maintaining consistent bedtimes and waking times, even on weekends. Throwing off this cycle can be as disruptive to migraine sufferers as jet lag might be to frequent travelers. It's about creating predictability for the brain, aligning our internal clock, and reducing unexpected fluctuations that might trigger migraines.

The role of light in sleep hygiene can't be understated. While natural daylight exposure boosts our alertness during the day, reducing exposure to blue light from screens at night is crucial. This helps encourage the natural production of melatonin, the hormone responsible for regulating sleep. Migraines can be particularly sensitive to light changes, so reducing artificial light exposure can be doubly beneficial.

An often neglected aspect of sleep hygiene is the pre-sleep routine. Engaging in calming activities like reading a book or practicing gentle yoga can signal the brain that it's time to wind down. Avoiding stimulating activities such as checking emails or scrolling through news feeds—can make a remarkable difference. These routines prepare both mind and body for a more restful state, and over time, they might link these habits to improved migraine triggers.

Environmental factors play an integral role. Investing in a comfortable mattress and pillow can reduce physical discomfort that might lead to restless nights. It's equally important to keep the bedroom cool and quiet to further promote relaxation. Sensory disturbances, such as noise and uncomfortable room temperature, are known migraine triggers, making them pertinent concerns for those crafting optimal sleep conditions.

But what about caffeine? It's a double-edged sword. While caffeine can sometimes alleviate acute migraine symptoms, it can also disrupt sleep if consumed later in the day. Therefore, understanding your body's unique tolerance and recognizing the timing of caffeine intake become essential parts of personalized sleep hygiene practices. It all boils down to balance and understanding your body's needs.

Regular physical activity is another cornerstone. Exercise can promote deeper sleep cycles and reduce stress levels, both of which are beneficial in managing migraines. However, the timing and intensity of exercise matter. Vigorous exercise close to bedtime might be counterproductive, making moderate and early workouts a better choice.

Maintaining a migraine journal can be enlightening. By recording sleep patterns and identifying nights that precede migraine attacks, individuals can discern specific changes or practices that might need adjustment. This self-monitoring leads to a more tailored approach to sleep hygiene, addressing personal triggers, and optimizing nightly routines. It's akin to becoming one's own sleep detective.

For some, anxiety around getting enough sleep can actually impair sleep. If you're worrying about falling asleep to prevent migraines, it can create a vicious cycle. Cognitive Behavioral Therapy for Insomnia (CBT-I) teaches strategies to manage the worry and shift focus away from the distress surrounding sleep challenges. Such psychological interventions hold great promise for those whose migrainous thresholds are tightly linked with sleep concerns.

To summarize, embracing sleep hygiene is a journey toward discovering what works best for your unique needs. It's an invitation to experiment with different approaches, listening attentively to how your body and mind respond. By cementing these practices as part of your daily life, you not only tackle one major trigger head-on but also inch closer to a lifestyle where migraines don't hold absolute power over your day.

So, as you integrate these sleep hygiene tactics into your daily routine, remember that each adjustment brings you a step nearer to reclaiming wellness, turning nights that once held apprehension into opportunities for healing and renewal. Sleep is not merely the absence of wakefulness but a foundational component of our holistic health, especially for those navigating the complexities of migraines.

Creating a Sleep-Friendly Environment

When dealing with migraines, a sleep-friendly environment can serve as a vital sanctuary to soothe and potentially stave off debilitating attacks. It's no secret that inadequate or erratic sleep can trigger migraines for many sufferers. The secret, then, lies in crafting an atmosphere conducive to uninterrupted and restorative slumber. Let's explore how you can transform your sleep space into a haven of rest and recovery.

First, consider the environment's foundation: temperature and light. A cool, dark room is optimal for encouraging sleep. Temperature regulation often falls by the wayside, but it's paramount. Aim for a bedroom temperature between 60 and 67 degrees Fahrenheit. This range supports the body's natural cool-down instinct that occurs as you drift towards sleep. Utilize blackout curtains to block out external light sources, such as street lights or early morning sun, ensuring your room remains blissfully dimmed. Blackout curtains are a small investment that can yield substantial dividends in seamless sleep.

It's not just about blocking out the light; minimizing noise is another crucial aspect. For those sensitive to sound, even the faintest noise can disrupt sleep architecture, inviting migraines. White noise machines, fans, or soothing sound apps can mask jarring interruptions. These tools create a consistent sound environment, which can significantly reduce sleep disruptions and help lull you into a deeper sleep cycle. Consider earplugs if shared walls or city sounds are part and parcel of your dwelling.

The bed itself — a personal haven within your room — deserves careful attention. Invest in a quality mattress that offers the right balance of support and comfort for your body. Your spine's alignment is crucial, as poor posture during sleep can lead to tension headaches, which can sometimes trigger migraines. Memory foam or hybrid mattresses could be worth considering. Additionally, choose pillows that support your head and neck properly. Pillows are not meant to last a lifetime; evaluate their condition every few years.

Bedding materials can influence the quality of your sleep as well. Select breathable, natural fibers like cotton or bamboo, which allow for proper airflow and can help maintain a comfortable body temperature throughout the night. Hypoallergenic options are beneficial if you're prone to allergies, which can exacerbate headaches.

Diving into the psychology of sleep preparation, we must consider the role of color schemes within the bedroom. Soft, muted hues— think blues, lavenders, and greens—promote relaxation. These colors can calm the mind, setting the stage for sleep. Brighter colors might energize and distract, whereas darker tones can create a sense of coziness and security which is invaluable for restful sleep.

Technology, though a marvel of modern life, could be an insidious sleep-stealer. Research shows that the blue light emitted by screens interferes with the production of melatonin, a hormone responsible for regulating sleep cycles. It's best to keep devices out of the bedroom whenever possible. Turn off screens at least an hour before bed, or use night modes and blue light filters if screen time in the evenings is unavoidable. Consider old-school methods for relaxation, like reading a book or engaging in gentle stretches before bedtime.

Finally, let's not forget the power of scent. Aromatherapy diffused into the bedroom air could enhance your sleep quality. Lavender and chamomile are renowned for their calming properties and are widely used to aid sleep. An essential oil diffuser releasing these scents into the room might help you drift into dreamland more easily, without harmful side effects.

Creating a sanctuary requires a holistic approach, acknowledging that sleep quality can be a robust ally against migraines. Everything from the bedding to the color of the walls, from the sounds around you to the scents you breathe in, can contribute to a space that invites restorative sleep. As crucial as these external factors may be, remember the internal ones as well: approach sleep with a peaceful mind, freed from the burdens of the day. Meditation or deep-breathing exercises before bed can help ease tension and prepare you for what we might truly call the perfect night's sleep.

Migraines don't have to dictate your nights. Transforming your bedroom into a sleep sanctuary empowers you, turning rest into a vital component of managing and mitigating migraine episodes. Through thoughtful adjustments, you can reclaim nights of peace and days of renewed energy.

Chapter 16:
Hormones and Migraines

For many migraine sufferers, hormonal fluctuations are the hidden puppeteers, pulling strings that can exacerbate or even trigger debilitating attacks. Understanding the dynamic relationship between hormones and migraines is crucial in the quest for relief. As estrogen levels ebb and flow—most notably during menstrual cycles, pregnancy, and menopause—they can significantly influence migraine patterns. Women, in particular, often notice a correlation between these hormonal shifts and the frequency or intensity of their headaches. Empowered by this knowledge, it's possible to anticipate and manage hormonal triggers with strategies such as tracking hormonal cycles, considering birth control options, and exploring medical treatments that stabilize hormone levels. The goal is to regain control and reduce the impact of hormones on your daily life, transforming what might seem like an insurmountable challenge into an opportunity for self-awareness and proactive management.

Understanding Hormonal Impact

Hormones, those tiny messengers in our body, wield an incredible influence over a multitude of physiological processes, and migraines are no exception. For many, hormonal fluctuations can set off migraine attacks, transforming what might otherwise be a regular day into one clouded with pain. Understanding these hormonal impacts is crucial for both managing and predicting migraine occurrences, as this knowledge can empower sufferers to navigate their condition more effectively.

One of the most common times people experience hormonal migraines is during menstruation. Often termed "menstrual migraines," these occur around the onset of a woman's period, thanks in large part to the dramatic drop in estrogen levels. It's estimated that up to 60% of women who suffer from migraines report a significant increase in attacks related to their menstrual cycle. This isn't just anecdotal; research supports the relationship between falling estrogen levels and migraine onset.

But it's not just menstruation that plays a role. Hormonal changes during pregnancy and menopause can also influence migraine patterns. During pregnancy, some women experience a reduction in migraines, especially during the second and third trimesters, due to stable, elevated hormone levels. Yet, others continue to suffer or even experience their first migraines during pregnancy, underscoring the complex nature of hormonal effects. As for menopause, the fluctuating hormone levels can either exacerbate or alleviate migraine symptoms, with experiences varying from person to person.

Beyond the gendered hormones like estrogen and progesterone, other hormones such as cortisol, thyroxine, and insulin can affect migraines. Stress, for instance, can increase levels of cortisol, a hormone that might contribute to triggering or intensifying symptoms. Thyroid imbalances, whether hypothyroidism or hyperthyroidism, influence migraine frequency and intensity, given the thyroid's role in metabolism and energy regulation. Blood sugar regulation, driven by insulin, also plays its part; fluctuations here can lead to heightened migraine activity, particularly if blood sugar drops too low.

The interaction between hormones and neurotransmitters further complicates the picture. Serotonin, a well-known neurotransmitter in the world of migraines, is significantly affected by hormonal changes.

Estrogen helps modulate serotonin levels, and as estrogen levels vary, so do serotonin levels. This can partly explain the timing of migraines in relation to menstrual cycles, as lower estrogen means lower serotonin, potentially leading to an increased incidence of migraines.

Understanding these connections isn't just an academic exercise; it offers practical significance. By recognizing these patterns, migraine sufferers can work to mitigate the effects. Hormone-triggered migraines, for example, might be managed with hormonal therapies or lifestyle adjustments aimed at stabilizing these swings. Some women find relief by using hormonal birth control methods to maintain consistent hormone levels, though this approach isn't without its own set of considerations and should be discussed at length with a healthcare provider.

Diet and lifestyle can also be adjusted to help manage hormonal impacts. For insulin-related issues, maintaining a balanced diet with regular meals can help stabilize blood sugar levels, potentially reducing the frequency of migraines. Regular physical activity, sufficient hydration, and adequate sleep are beneficial in maintaining overall hormonal balance, though they require personalization to suit individual needs and triggers.

Moreover, tracking hormonal patterns can illuminate trends that may not be immediately obvious. Keeping a detailed migraine journal, which correlates migraines with menstrual cycles, stress levels, or dietary changes, can highlight hormonal impacts. This self-awareness allows for better communication with healthcare providers, making it easier to tailor a therapeutic approach that fits the individual's unique hormonal profile.

Ultimately, understanding the hormonal impact on migraines involves patience and a willingness to observe one's own body and its responses. This journey is personal, unique to each individual, reflecting not only the complexity of migraines but also the intricate, intertwining nature of our bodily systems. Through this understanding, those impacted by migraines can find new avenues to explore in their quest for relief, equipping themselves with knowledge that both empowers and inspires.

Managing Hormonal Triggers

Hormones play a crucial role in migraines, especially for those who find their headache patterns aligning with the ebb and flow of their body's hormonal cycle. For many, these hormones are not just another trigger but the most potent one of all. Understanding and managing hormonal influences can empower individuals to take active steps in mitigating migraine risks associated with hormonal changes. This is most commonly observed in individuals who experience migraines before or during menstruation, known as menstrual migraines, but hormones can also impact those who are pregnant, going through menopause, or using hormone-based therapies.

Identifying the particular hormonal changes that precipitate migraines is the first step towards management. Many find that keeping a meticulous migraine journal can reveal patterns connected to their menstrual cycle, pregnancy, or menopausal stage. By tracking the timing, severity, and frequency of migraines alongside hormonal fluctuations, individuals may begin to see correlations that had previously gone unnoticed. As patterns emerge, it's vital to share these findings with healthcare providers to tailor a management plan that best suits their hormonal cycle.

An effective strategy to manage hormonal triggers is stabilizing hormonal fluctuations. This can be achieved through both lifestyle changes and medical interventions. For some, hormonal contraceptives can help by flattening the peaks and troughs of hormonal variations. However, this is a complex decision and must be made in consultation with healthcare professionals, balancing the benefits of migraine prevention against potential side effects. Non-hormonal options like magnesium supplements and vitamin B2 may also play a part in alleviating migraine frequency or severity around hormonal shifts.

Lifestyle adjustments are another powerful tool in managing hormonal migraine triggers. Regular sleep patterns, a balanced diet rich in anti-inflammatory foods, and consistent physical activity can enhance overall well-being and potentially ease migraine occurrence. Stress is another significant factor that can exacerbate hormone-triggered migraines, making stress management techniques such as yoga, meditation, and deep-breathing exercises valuable complements to other treatments.

Acupuncture and biofeedback have shown promises as alternative therapies for managing migraines, including those influenced by hormones. These approaches focus on restoring balance to the body's systems and can serve as adjuncts to traditional medical treatments. Some find that integrating mind-body practices helps create a sense of control and reduces the tension that often accompanies life's hormonal shifts.

For those who experience migraines tied closely to menstrual cycles, predictable prevention strategies can make a substantial difference. This might involve taking migraine-preventative medications just before and during their menstruation period. Non-steroidal anti-inflammatory drugs (NSAIDs) are commonly prescribed for this purpose, though other options include triptans or even hormonal treatments as mentioned before.

Frequent communication with healthcare providers is crucial in navigating the complexities of hormone-related migraines. Every person reacts differently to hormones and medications, and what works for one might not work for another. A customized plan, crafted with input from both patient and provider, increases the likelihood of a successful outcome in reducing migraine attacks.

While hormonal changes present a challenging component in migraine management, staying informed about new medical insights and treatments is key. Research continues to uncover more about the mechanisms by which hormones influence migraines, and staying updated allows you to take advantage of evolving therapies and strategies. Support groups, both online and in-person, can provide communal wisdom from others who share your experience and can offer encouragement and tips that supplement medical advice.

In essence, by understanding your body's hormonal rhythms and how they intersect with migraine attacks, you gain powerful insights into how to better manage your symptoms. Balancing hormones may require dedicated effort and patience, but it can lead to a significant reduction in migraine frequency and intensity, ultimately improving quality of life.

Chapter 17:
Migraine Myths and Facts

Migraines often come burdened with misconceptions that can hinder effective management and understanding. One prevalent myth is that migraines are simply bad headaches, but those who suffer know they're far more complex and debilitating. These neurological events don't just affect the head; they can disrupt vision, balance, and even speech, carrying an invisible weight that extends beyond pain. Contrary to popular belief, migraines aren't always a result of stress or diet, and they're not purely psychosomatic. In fact, scientific research has shown that genetic, environmental, and even hormonal factors can play significant roles. By understanding these evidence-based facts, sufferers and supporters alike can shift their perspectives, fostering compassion and creating informed approaches to tackling the challenges of living with migraines. Dispelling these myths empowers individuals, offering a clearer path to effective symptom management and an improved quality of life.

Debunking Common Myths

The world of migraines is fraught with misconceptions, often perpetuated by well-meaning individuals who lack a thorough understanding of the condition. These myths can lead to an overwhelming sense of isolation for sufferers, making it crucial to dissect and dispel them. Doing so not only provides clarity but also empowers those affected, giving them the confidence to seek appropriate treatment and support.

One common myth is the belief that migraines are just severe headaches. This misconception is damaging because it minimizes the multifaceted nature of the condition. A migraine is a complex neurological disorder, characterized by a range of symptoms that can include debilitating pain, nausea, visual disturbances, and sensitivity to light and sound, among others. Understanding the full scope of a migraine attack helps dismantle this myth and validates the experiences of those enduring it.

Another pervasive myth suggests that migraines are simply a result of stress or that they occur because someone can't handle stress effectively. While stress can undoubtedly trigger migraines, it's a gross oversimplification to attribute the condition solely to stress management issues. The reality is that migraines have a myriad of triggers, including hormonal changes, dietary factors, environmental stimuli, and genetic predispositions. Recognizing this complexity is vital in shifting the blame away from the individual and towards the condition.

People often believe migraines are exclusive to women, which is not the case. While it's true women are three times more likely to experience migraines, men and even children can suffer from them as well. This myth can lead to underdiagnosis and inadequate treatment for male sufferers, adding yet another layer of difficulty in managing the condition. Acknowledging that migraines don't discriminate by gender is crucial for equitable care.

There is also a common belief that migraines aren't a serious health issue because they don't cause any permanent damage. While it's true that migraines don't directly cause brain damage, their impact on an individual's quality of life and daily functioning can be profound. Chronic migraines, in particular, can lead to significant impairment, with individuals losing productivity at work or school and often experiencing mental health challenges such as depression and anxiety.

Another myth claims that if a treatment works for one person, it will work for anyone. In reality, migraines are highly individualized, and what relieves symptoms for one person might not do the same for another. This can be incredibly frustrating for sufferers searching for relief. Effective management often requires a tailored approach that may include various combinations of medications, lifestyle changes, and alternative therapies.

The idea that "migraines can be cured" is a particularly misleading myth that sets unrealistic expectations. While it's possible to manage and reduce the frequency and severity of migraines, they cannot be completely eradicated or cured. Educating sufferers about the chronic nature of migraines and focusing on evidence-based management strategies helps to set realistic goals and expectations, guiding them towards a life where migraines play a less prominent role.

Some individuals mistakenly believe that migraine attacks can always be avoided if one is vigilant enough. Although identifying triggers and making lifestyle adjustments can significantly reduce the occurrence of migraine episodes, completely avoiding them is not always feasible. This myth can lead to unnecessary guilt and self-blame when attacks occur despite best efforts. Emphasizing the importance of self-compassion and understanding can help mitigate these feelings.

It's also often thought that people with migraines exaggerate their symptoms or use them as an excuse to avoid responsibilities. This myth undermines the legitimate and often severe impact that migraines have on sufferers' lives. It's crucial to foster a cultural shift towards empathy and understanding, recognizing that migraines are not just a "get-out-of-jail-free card" but a genuine medical condition requiring attention and care.

In conclusion, debunking these common myths is essential in changing the narrative surrounding migraines. This process not only dispels falsehoods but also paves the way for more informed discussions and better support systems. By spreading awareness and understanding, we can equip both sufferers and their support networks with the tools needed to manage migraines more effectively, ultimately enhancing the quality of life for those affected.

As these myths unravel, the real conversations about migraines can begin, focusing on evidence-based facts, individualized treatment plans, and a compassionate approach that respects the chronic nature of the condition. It is only through dismantling these misconceptions that we can hope to alleviate not just the physical burden of migraines, but also the emotional and societal ones that accompany them.

Evidence-Based Facts

Migraines have long been a source of mystery and misunderstanding, but modern research has provided us with a clearer picture of this complex condition. With advancements in neuroimaging, genetic studies, and clinical trials, we've gained significant insights into the biological basis of migraines. These insights demystify misconceptions and offer evidence-based truths, empowering those who suffer from migraines to take a proactive role in managing their condition.

First and foremost, migraines are not "just a headache." They are a neurological disorder characterized by a variety of symptoms, including intense head pain, sensitivity to light and sound, nausea, and in some cases, visual disturbances known as auras. Studies using functional MRI and PET scans have revealed that migraines are linked to physiological changes in blood flow and chemical activity in the brain, implicating areas such as the hypothalamus, thalamus, and brainstem.

Dr. Felix Fielding

Importantly, genetics play a role in migraines, although they aren't the sole cause. Research has identified certain genetic markers that increase susceptibility to migraines, providing evidence that they can run in families. While genetic predisposition can't be altered, understanding one's genetic risk can inform treatment strategies and lifestyle modifications to help prevent attacks.

The relationship between migraines and vascular phenomena has been re-evaluated over the years. Once thought to be solely caused by changes in blood vessel dilation and constriction, it's now understood that neurological pathways and neurotransmitter imbalances are crucial players in triggering migraine episodes. The role of serotonin, a key neurotransmitter, has been extensively documented, with decreased serotonin levels during migraines potentially leading to the dilation of blood vessels, thereby contributing to the throbbing pain characteristic of the disorder.

There is also compelling evidence that migraines involve hyperexcitability of the cerebral cortex. This hyperexcitability can cause neurons to fire more easily, triggering the sensory disturbances often experienced during an aura and the subsequent cascade of symptoms. Understanding this mechanism has paved the way for targeted treatments that focus on stabilizing neuronal activity, thus reducing the frequency and severity of attacks.

Evidence also supports the notion that migraines are influenced by hormonal fluctuations, particularly in women. Hormonal changes during menstrual cycles, pregnancy, and menopause can exacerbate migraine symptoms, implicating hormones such as estrogen in the process. This evidence underscores the importance of a personalized approach to treatment that takes hormonal influences into account.

Lifestyle factors are frequently highlighted in managing migraines, and scientific research supports the effectiveness of certain adjustments. Regular sleep patterns, adequate hydration, and maintaining stable blood sugar levels have been shown to reduce the frequency and intensity of migraines. Incorporating these strategies, backed by empirical evidence, empowers individuals to take an active role in their migraine management.

Stress and emotional well-being also affect migraines, with studies indicating that stress management techniques can significantly reduce migraine occurrences. The evidence supports practices like meditation, cognitive behavioral therapy, and mindfulness as beneficial adjuncts to traditional medical treatments. By addressing the psychological components associated with migraines, individuals can experience an overall improvement in their quality of life.

Moreover, the benefits of regular physical activity for migraine sufferers are well-documented in scientific literature. Aerobic exercises have been shown to release endorphins, natural pain-killers that alleviate migraine pain and improve mood. Though it may seem counterintuitive, consistent, moderate exercise can indeed be a protective factor against migraines, helping prevent onset and reduce the severity of episodes.

Dietary connections to migraines are another area where evidence provides practical guidance. Certain foods and additives are known triggers for some migraine sufferers. Empirical studies suggest that keeping a food journal and identifying personal dietary triggers can be a critical step in managing the condition. This proactive approach allows individuals to avoid triggers and potentially reduce the frequency of their migraines.

The pharmacological landscape for treating migraines has expanded significantly, thanks to rigorously tested and approved medications. Triptans, a class of drugs specifically developed for migraines, are designed to target serotonin receptors and have been demonstrated to be effective in aborting migraine attacks when taken early. This represents a significant advancement in migraine treatment, moving beyond general pain relief to address the specific pathways involved in migraine pathophysiology.

Chronic migraines, affecting a small but significant subset of migraineurs, have specific treatment guidelines rooted in evidence. Preventive medications, often used daily, have been shown in studies to drastically reduce the number of days people suffer from migraines. These treatments aim not just at symptom relief but at altering the disease's course, providing hope for those affected.

Finally, while the interplay of these factors can be complex, a multifaceted approach is vital in treatment. Tailored treatment plans combining lifestyle adjustments, dietary awareness, pharmacological interventions, and stress management techniques are often the most successful. By rigorously applying evidence-based knowledge, migraine sufferers can achieve better control over their condition, helping them to lead fuller, more comfortable lives.

In conclusion, evidence-based research has demystified many elements of migraines, providing clear pathways to effective management and treatment. This knowledge dispels myths and replaces them with empowering facts, confirming the real, tangible nature of migraines and offering concrete tools to improve life for those who experience them regularly. Armed with these insights, sufferers, family members, and healthcare providers alike can approach migraines with informed strategies, moving towards a world where the burden of this condition is significantly diminished.

Chapter 18:
Parental Guidance on Migraines

As a parent navigating the rough waters of childhood migraines, the balance between providing comfort and implementing practical strategies can feel overwhelming. Yet, with the right guidance, you can play a pivotal role in your child's journey toward migraine management. Understandably, your child's experience of pain is not only a physical battle but an emotional one too; thus, your support is essential. Collaborate with educators to ensure academic accommodations and understand the powerful impact of open lines of communication with healthcare professionals. By consistently advocating for your child's needs and fostering an environment of empathy, you create a foundation for effective migraine management. Empowering your child with coping mechanisms early on can bolster resilience, turning these challenging moments into opportunities for growth and understanding. Together, step by step, you can navigate this journey and cultivate an atmosphere where your child feels heard, supported, and ready to face each day with confidence.

Supporting a Child with Migraines

Helping a child who experiences migraines can be a challenging and emotional journey for any parent. Witnessing their young one go through the pain, discomfort, and often confusion associated with these intense headaches can feel overwhelming. But with guidance, understanding, and patience, parents can play a pivotal role in managing their child's condition effectively, ensuring that the child continues to lead a fulfilling and active life.

Migraines in children can manifest differently than in adults. Recognizing the specific symptoms that your child might exhibit is the first step toward offering effective support. These symptoms could range from throbbing pain on one side of the head to sensitivity to light, sound, or even smell. Some children may experience nausea or vomiting, while others might appear unusually quiet or withdrawn. Understanding these signs is crucial because timely identification can lead to quicker relief and prevention of severity.

Start by creating an open, non-judgmental space where your child feels comfortable discussing their experiences. Encouraging them to articulate what they feel can not only give you insights into their condition but also helps your child become more self-aware, increasing their ability to manage symptoms independently. You might hear stories of how certain foods, bright lights, or particular activities precede a migraine. These narratives are invaluable. They're not just reflections of your child's experiences, but also potential clues pointing toward specific triggers that can be managed or avoided.

Incorporating a migraine journal for your child can be immensely helpful. This tool allows you both to track patterns and common triggers systematically. Together, you can note episodes, evaluate current coping strategies, and adjust them if necessary. Over time, this practice can reveal valuable insights, enabling more precise and personalized management strategies. It's a dynamic process—what worked yesterday may not work tomorrow—and a journal helps you keep track of this evolving understanding.

Next, work on adapting the child's environment to meet their unique needs. This could range from ensuring that their room offers a calm and quiet space to learning how to moderate lighting levels and control noise. Schools can also be made more accommodating. Inform teachers and administrators about your child's condition and collaborate with them on devising backup plans for migraine days— whether it's allowing for short rests in a quiet space or modified workloads. Educational support is crucial to make sure that migraines don't interfere significantly with learning and school participation.

Adjustment of daily routines can also make a significant difference. Regular sleep patterns, balanced nutrition, and adequate hydration may reduce the frequency and severity of migraine episodes. Encourage your child to partake in physical activities that are within their comfort zone. The endorphins released during exercise can act as natural pain relievers, as long as the activity doesn't become a trigger itself.

Integrating stress management techniques tailored to children can be beneficial as well. Simple breathing exercises, gentle yoga, or guided meditations can help them manage stress, a common migraine trigger. Teaching these skills early gives children tools they can carry into adulthood, promoting long-term well-being.

Working closely with healthcare providers can unlock additional support. Pediatric neurologists or headache specialists can offer targeted treatments and medications that might relieve symptoms when they strike. Regular visits help to adapt these strategies as your child grows and their needs shift. They can also introduce alternative therapies like acupuncture, known to provide relief for some pediatric migraine sufferers, although these should be discussed in detail with a healthcare professional before being implemented.

As your child learns to navigate the social world, they might encounter situations where explaining their migraines becomes necessary. Role-playing scenarios at home can equip them with the language and confidence to communicate their needs effectively, whether it's asking a teacher for a quiet space or explaining to friends why they need to sit out from certain activities. This knowledge empowers them, builds resilience, and reduces the anxiety often associated with social interactions.

A crucial part of support is emotional backing. Recognize the emotional toll that chronic pain can have on a child. Encourage open dialogues about feelings and anxieties related to migraines. This not only fosters trust but strengthens the child's emotional resilience. Sometimes, professional counseling or therapy might be necessary, providing a safe avenue for children to explore and express deeper fears or frustrations.

Finally, as a parent, don't neglect your own emotional needs. Supporting a child with a chronic condition can be taxing. Reach out to support groups or online forums where other parents share similar experiences. This network not only offers emotional solace but can also provide practical tips and novel solutions you've not tried yet. Remember, your strength and well-being directly influence your child's ability to manage their own challenges.

Supporting a child through migraines is an ongoing journey, requiring nuanced observation, adaptation, and endless patience. But armed with knowledge, open communication, and strategic planning, parents can not only ease their child's journey through this complex condition but also instill in them a sense of agency and confidence that transcends the episodic pain of migraines.

Educational Support

Dealing with migraines is challenging enough, but when it afflicts children, it can feel downright overwhelming. This makes educational support not only beneficial but essential. Migraines can impact a child's daily school life, affecting their focus, attendance, and performance. To navigate this, parents, teachers, and support staff need to collaborate to ensure a supportive learning environment.

Understanding the educational challenges faced by children with migraines begins with recognizing the symptoms. They often experience severe headaches, nausea, and sensitivity to light or sound, which can make classroom environments uncomfortable or even unbearable. Frequent migraines may lead to absences that disrupt learning, causing a ripple effect in a child's academic progress. To mitigate these issues, it's vital to establish an open line of communication with your child's school.

First, parents should inform teachers and school administrators about their child's condition. Providing them with comprehensive information about migraines, along with specific triggers and symptoms relevant to the child can lead to a more empathetic approach in handling the child's needs. Schools often have protocols in place for managing health conditions, but each child's experience with migraines is unique, requiring personalized adjustments.

Supporting a child with migraines in school may involve creating a tailored plan, such as a 504 Plan or Individualized Education Program (IEP), if applicable. These plans are crucial as they formalize certain accommodations like allowing extra time for assignments and tests, the ability to leave the classroom when feeling unwell, or having a quiet place to rest when symptoms arise. It's essential that parents work with educators to determine what accommodations will be most beneficial.

Additionally, educating school staff about the importance of migraine awareness can make a difference. Many educators may not fully understand how debilitating migraines can be. Organizing informational sessions or providing resource materials can build a more supportive school culture. When teachers understand the potential impact on learning, they are more likely to be compassionate and accommodating.

Parents should also encourage their children to self-advocate whenever possible. Teaching children how to communicate their needs and when to request help plays a vital role in their growing independence. Encouraging them to speak with teachers directly about their condition can help foster confidence and reduce intimidation surrounding their health. It's beneficial for children to learn when to take breaks, use stress management techniques, or request specific classroom adjustments.

Outside the school environment, consider integrating technology that supports educational goals. Various apps and online resources offer tools for organizing assignments, managing time, and developing effective study strategies. Technology can assist children in staying on top of their work when they're physically absent from school.

Moreover, fostering a dialogue between school counselors and healthcare providers may provide fresh insights and strategies for management. Collaboration ensures that the child's needs are met holistically, respecting both their educational and health requirements. Sharing ideas between professionals might lead to novel approaches that work for your child.

It's also important to consider the emotional and social aspects of educational support. Migraine sufferers, especially children, may feel isolated or different from peers. Encourage participation in school activities where feasible, enabling social interactions that build a sense of community and support. Engaging with peers helps reduce the stigma associated with health conditions like migraines.

Finally, keep in mind that adjusting to migraines in the educational context is a continuous process. Reevaluate the accommodations and strategies regularly and make necessary changes. As children grow, their academic demands and their ways of interacting with the world evolve, and so should the support structures around them.

Empowering children with knowledge about their health condition is a cornerstone of managing migraines. When equipped with understanding and tools to succeed, children aren't just surviving their educational experience—they're thriving within it. By integrating educational support strategies, we lay a foundation not just for academic success but for a well-rounded, resilient individual who's well-prepared to deal with life's inevitable challenges.

Chapter 19:
Migraine Devices and Technology

In the realm of migraine management, technology has emerged as a formidable ally. From wearable devices that track and analyze migraine patterns through real-time data to innovative applications designed to provide immediate relief and comprehensive management strategies, these advancements offer a beacon of hope. Wearable tech, like smart headbands and neurostimulators, enables users to detect early warning signs and act swiftly to prevent full-blown attacks. Meanwhile, mobile apps have become indispensable, offering features that range from tracking symptoms and medications to sensory input for relaxation and behavioral modifications. These tools not only empower sufferers with immediate actions but also deepen their understanding through analytics, fostering a proactive approach to their health. Embracing these technologies can transform how one navigates the challenges of living with migraines, paving the way to a life less overshadowed by uncertainty and pain.

Wearable Tech for Monitoring

Migraine sufferers know all too well how challenging it can be to predict when the next debilitating episode will strike. The unpredictability not only affects daily plans but also one's quality of life. Fortunately, advances in wearable technology are paving the way for improved migraine management, offering a glimpse of hope for those seeking a way to monitor and potentially prevent attacks. These innovations merge technology with health insights, creating new possibilities for tracking and understanding migraines like never before.

One of the greatest advantages of wearable tech is its ability to gather real-time data seamlessly and unobtrusively. Devices like smartwatches and headbands equipped with sensors are not just limited to counting steps or monitoring heart rates anymore—they're evolving into specialized tools capable of tracking physiological changes that might precede migraine attacks. By monitoring changes in skin temperature, heart rate variability, and even brain activity, wearables can alert users to potential migraine triggers long before symptoms become apparent.

But why is continuous monitoring important? For many, migraines are triggered by subtle changes that are hard to notice without constant vigilance. Wearable devices, by providing consistent monitoring, capture variations that might escape notice during periodic checkups. This means that wearables can help establish patterns related to lifestyle choices, stress levels, and environmental factors, helping sufferers better understand their own unique triggers and potentially avoid them.

Imagine having the ability to receive a notification warning of an impending migraine attack. This is not science fiction; it's increasingly within reach. Certain wearables can already connect to smartphone apps that analyze patterns, detect anomalies, and even predict the likelihood of a migraine occurring. Users can then take preventive measures, whether that means taking prescribed medication, retreating to a quiet space, or employing stress-reduction techniques.

The ability to sync data from wearables with migraine journals and apps creates a powerful synergy. Many sufferers already use migraine journals to track symptoms, triggers, and treatments—a crucial practice outlined in the chapter on migraine journals. Wearables enhance this process by providing objective data. Users no longer rely solely on memory or subjective experiences. Instead, they can verify their personal insights with hard data, leading to more informed decisions and discussions with healthcare providers.

Moreover, this data can be shared with healthcare providers, transforming the doctor-patient relationship into a more collaborative partnership. Physicians can use the comprehensive data from wearables to detect trends and refine treatment plans more effectively. This level of detailed information enables healthcare professionals to provide personalized advice, honing in on specific factors that contribute to an individual's migraines, which could otherwise be overlooked or unknown.

The design and comfort of wearables also play a crucial role in their effectiveness. No one wants a device that's cumbersome or draws too much attention—especially when enduring a migraine. Manufacturers are increasingly aware of this, ensuring wearables are lightweight, discreet, and comfortable to wear for extended periods. Advances in battery technology and energy efficiency further ensure these devices can maintain functionality over the long periods needed for effective monitoring.

Despite the abundance of benefits, there are challenges that wearable tech currently faces. The accuracy of wearable monitoring technology is an ongoing area of development, with some devices still in early experimental stages. There's also the consideration of data privacy and the importance of ensuring users' health information remains secure. These are valid concerns, but as technology continues to improve, many of these hurdles are being reduced, and users can expect increasingly reliable and privacy-respecting solutions.

For those living with migraines, wearable technology offers a beacon of hope, assisting in the quest for a life less controlled by unexpected pain. As technology advances, the dream of seamlessly integrating lifestyle and health data for better migraine management becomes increasingly achievable. In the journey towards improved personal wellness, these devices add an important tool to the migraine management toolkit, simultaneously empowering users with more control over their condition.

The journey of managing migraines is deeply personal, and wearable tech represents a remarkable step forward in understanding and potentially mitigating the impact of this condition. While it may not be a cure, it certainly offers a promising way to navigate and manage the storms that migraines present, providing insights and information that were previously unattainable. Ultimately, these technologies are not just gadgets, but companions in our health journeys, guiding us towards achieving a fuller, more informed understanding of our bodies' rhythms.

Apps for Managing Symptoms

The realm of digital technology has woven itself into every corner of modern life, offering innovative solutions to age-old problems. For migraine sufferers, apps designed to manage symptoms can be a true lifeline, providing tools and resources that offer immediate relief, long-term management strategies, or simply a better understanding of one's condition. With a vast array of options available, finding the right app can feel overwhelming, yet the potential benefits make the journey worthwhile.

Apps for managing migraine symptoms generally fall into a few categories. Some focus on tracking and predicting symptoms, helping users identify triggers and patterns over time. These apps often allow individuals to log migraine occurrences, noting factors such as diet, sleep, stress, and even weather conditions. By analyzing this data, users can start recognizing the unique patterns that might lead to their migraines, giving them crucial insights into prevention.

Others act as virtual coaches, providing real-time guidance on how to mitigate the impact of migraines once they begin. These might include guided meditation sessions, breathing exercises, or on-demand advice for symptom relief. For many, simply having structured support readily available on their phone can reduce the stress and anxiety often accompanying a migraine episode.

The predictive capabilities of some apps have advanced significantly in recent years. By employing machine learning algorithms, these apps can anticipate the potential onset of a migraine before noticeable symptoms occur. These predictions are based on historical data and subtle changes in the user's reported lifestyle habits, allowing for preemptive measures to be taken. Early intervention can significantly reduce the intensity and duration of migraines, emphasizing the power of technology in proactive health management.

In addition to prediction and tracking, some apps facilitate connection to peer support networks. The isolation that can accompany chronic migraine conditions is daunting, but knowing others are going through the same can bring comfort. Community-based apps enable users to share experiences, tips, and encouragement, creating a sense of belonging that can be as therapeutic as any medication or treatment.

Privacy and security are paramount when using apps that deal with personal health information. Reputable apps typically have clear privacy policies and use encryption to protect user data. It's essential for users to familiarize themselves with these policies to feel confident that their sensitive information remains confidential.

Despite the variety and promise of migraine management apps, there are practical considerations to keep in mind. Not every app will suit every individual, and some trial and error may be necessary to find one that aligns with personal needs and preferences. Additionally, while apps can be an excellent tool for managing symptoms, they should complement, not replace, professional medical advice.

As the landscape of digital health continues to evolve, so too does the potential for apps to play a critical role in managing migraines. The convenience of having personalized, actionable advice and historical data at one's fingertips can empower individuals to take greater control of their health. By integrating these digital tools into their routine, migraine sufferers can find a measure of relief and understanding, transforming a once-overwhelming condition into one that is more predictable and manageable.

Ultimately, the choice of app should resonate with the user's lifestyle and specific needs, providing a seamless fit into their daily lives. Technology, when utilized effectively, not only helps in tackling immediate challenges but can also pave the way for more profound, long-lasting changes in managing migraines. In the dance between technology and health, those intricate apps developed for managing migraines are proving to be valuable partners in the journey to wellness.

Chapter 20:
Long-Term Strategies

As we delve into long-term strategies for managing migraines, it's essential to cultivate a personalized action plan that evolves with your unique journey. Recognizing the dynamic nature of migraines means setting realistic goals that accommodate life's inevitable shifts. This chapter encourages you to view management as a proactive, flexible process rather than a static checklist. Building on the solid foundation of understanding, lifestyle adjustments, and medical support discussed throughout this book, establish a sustainable regimen that seamlessly integrates into your everyday life. Empower yourself by harnessing the insights you've gained, and embrace a mindset of resilience and adaptation. Together, these strategies form a roadmap to not just manage, but transform your migraine experience into one that prioritizes well-being and enhances your quality of life.

Developing a Migraine Action Plan

Crafting a migraine action plan can transform your experience with migraines, turning moments of overwhelming pain into manageable and predictable events. An action plan is more than just a series of steps; it's a commitment to understanding your condition and using that knowledge to minimize its impact on your life. It's about reclaiming control when every migraine threatens to strip it away.

The first and perhaps most pivotal component of a migraine action plan is self-awareness. Understanding your specific migraine triggers is essential. While common triggers like stress, lack of sleep, or specific foods might be well documented, it'll be crucial to identify what precisely affects you. By keeping a detailed migraine journal over a period of time, you'll have the means to track potential triggers. Each migraine will leave behind footprints, patterns of change or static elements that can guide you in deciphering what needs to change.

Once you've identified the potential triggers, the next step is to establish avoidance and mitigation strategies tailored to your lifestyle. This might mean adjusting your diet, ensuring you stick to a consistent sleep schedule, or finding new ways to handle stress — elements thoroughly discussed elsewhere in this book. Tailoring your environment and habits to reduce exposure to known triggers is a proactive step in managing migraines long-term.

However, even with the best of preventative measures, migraines can break through your defenses. That's where understanding your treatment options comes in. An action plan should include a comprehensive list of medical treatments that have been identified as effective for your specific migraines. This might include over-the-counter medication that you've gauged to be effective, prescription treatments agreed upon with healthcare providers, or alternative therapies that offer symptom relief.

Having a treatment hierarchy can be immensely helpful when you feel a migraine approaching. This hierarchy could include immediate actions, like taking medication at the first sign of symptoms, followed by secondary measures such as a dark, quiet room or relaxation techniques. Relief can sometimes feel elusive, but knowing exactly what to do and when can bring a reassuring structure to moments of chaos.

Equally important is having a plan for when to seek additional medical help. It's vital to recognize when a migraine is beyond what your current plan can manage. Having thresholds — such as the occurrence of new symptoms or a change in headache volume or intensity — will enable you to know when it's time to seek further medical attention.

Communicating your action plan effectively with those around you is another crucial aspect. Family, friends, and workplaces play significant roles, and informing them of your strategies can foster a supportive environment. Share what signs indicate an approaching migraine and what they can do to assist or accommodate you in such times. This proactive communication can transform potential periods of vulnerability into times of shared understanding and support.

Your plan should also accommodate moments of reflection and adaptation. Migraines are not static, and neither should your strategies be. Regularly reviewing and updating your action plan allows it to evolve alongside your understanding and life changes. Periodic reassessment, possibly in collaboration with healthcare providers, will ensure that your plan remains effective and relevant.

In crafting and refining your migraine action plan, remember this: it's an ongoing journey. It requires patience, a willingness to learn, and importantly, a commitment to self-care. With each step forward, you're not just managing symptoms but actively enhancing the quality of your life. This empowerment fuels the resilience needed to live well despite chronic conditions.

Ultimately, a migraine action plan does more than offer a blueprint; it provides peace of mind. Knowing that you have a well-considered strategy can reduce anxiety and boost your confidence. As life's unpredictability interplays with migraines, a thoughtfully developed plan ensures you're as prepared as possible, equipping you to navigate both everyday and unforeseen challenges.

Setting Realistic Goals

Setting realistic goals is a cornerstone in the journey to understanding and managing migraines. It isn't about creating a dream scenario where migraines cease to exist, but rather establishing attainable milestones that empower and encourage continual progress. The path towards long-term relief is often challenging, filled with fluctuations and plateaus. Yet, creating achievable targets can provide direction and a sense of accomplishment, fostering a positive outlook even in the face of setbacks.

The first step in setting realistic goals is self-awareness. Begin by understanding your unique migraine triggers, symptoms, and the frequency and intensity of your attacks. Tracking these details is essential in formulating a practical strategy. This enables not just the identification of patterns, but also aids in preparing for potential disruptions, much like one might prepare for changes in the weather. A well-maintained migraine journal acts as a valuable tool here, offering insights that can guide decisions and goal-setting.

When establishing goals, pace yourself. Initially, it could be as simple as keeping a regular sleep schedule or reducing caffeine intake. Small steps build momentum and lay the foundation for more significant changes. Celebrate these small victories—they are the building blocks of larger achievements. These incremental goals serve to gradually adjust lifestyle habits, which in turn may reduce the frequency or severity of migraine attacks.

Building a strong support network is vital for staying on track. Share your goals with family, friends, and healthcare providers. This external support can provide motivation and accountability, making it easier to stick to your plans. Honest communication with those around you about your needs and challenges fosters an environment of understanding and compassion, which can significantly enhance your coping mechanisms.

Another critical aspect is flexibility. Migraines can be unpredictable, making rigid goals impractical and potentially discouraging. Incorporate adaptability into your goal-setting strategy. If you miss a target due to an unexpected migraine attack, acknowledge the setback and adjust your plan accordingly. Recognize that progress will not always be linear; there will be ups and downs, and that's okay. Flexibility ensures that you remain resilient, adapting your strategies to fit your current circumstances rather than giving up altogether.

Consider incorporating a variety of approaches in your goals, combining lifestyle changes, dietary adjustments, medical treatments, and stress management techniques. This multidimensional strategy acknowledges the complexity of migraines and allows for a more holistic approach. For example, committing to a daily meditation practice or integrating specific exercises suited for migraine sufferers can be both manageable and effective when combined with medical advice.

It's also helpful to set both short-term and long-term goals. Short-term goals are the actionable steps you can implement right away—like incorporating a new relaxation technique into your daily routine. Long-term goals might involve broader lifestyle changes, such as achieving a balanced diet tailored to your needs. Together, they create a roadmap that balances immediate relief with sustainable change, guiding you towards improved quality of life.

Remember to periodically review and reflect on your goals. This is not just about checking off boxes but understanding what strategies are working and which need refinement. Regular reflection helps maintain focus and motivation. It can also highlight successes that might otherwise go unnoticed, reinforcing your commitment and providing a clear picture of your journey.

In the context of developing your migraine action plan, realistic goal setting is about empowerment and taking control. It emphasizes your ability to make informed decisions about your health, fostering a proactive rather than reactive approach. By setting goals that are both challenging and attainable, you create a pathway to self-efficacy and resilience, essential traits in managing chronic conditions like migraines.

In closing, setting realistic goals is not just a task, but a mindset. It involves patience, perseverance, and the willingness to adapt. While the journey may seem daunting, each step forward is a testament to your strength and determination. Migraines needn't define your life or your limits. By setting realistic goals, you carve a path towards a future with more freedom and less pain, underpinned by the knowledge and empowerment to manage your condition effectively.

Chapter 21:
Mental Health and Migraines

In the intricate dance between mental health and migraines, understanding the deep, sometimes reciprocal, relationship between mind and body is crucial. For many, the presence of a migraine can fuel feelings of anxiety and depression, while existing mental health challenges may exacerbate migraine symptoms, creating a challenging cycle. This chapter explores how sensitive awareness of one's mental state can be instrumental in breaking this cycle. It's essential to recognize patterns in mood and emotional responses as potential indicators for impending migraines, spotlighting the importance of mental well-being. Effective management might involve seeking professional help or integrating mindfulness practices into daily routines to bolster resilience. Embracing therapy and possibly medication where needed can lend insight and provide relief, ultimately enhancing life quality for migraine sufferers. Cultivating a compassionate understanding toward oneself and others facing these challenges can transform this journey into one of empowerment and healing.

Addressing Anxiety and Depression

Migraines aren't just about the physical pain—they often bring along a heavy emotional toll. The link between mental health and migraines is well-documented, with anxiety and depression frequently accompanying the throbbing pain of a migraine attack. For those navigating the challenge of living with migraines, understanding and addressing these emotional burdens can be a transformative part of their journey.

It's not uncommon for migraine sufferers to feel a sense of dread leading up to a migraine. This anticipatory anxiety can exacerbate the condition, making it harder to manage the symptoms when they do appear. This cycle of anxiety and pain creates a feedback loop, wherein the stress of expecting a migraine builds and potentially triggers another attack. Recognizing this cycle is a key step in breaking it. The first step in mitigating these issues often lies in heightened self-awareness and proactive strategies aimed at self-compassion.

Depression also frequently shadows those with chronic migraines. The persistent, unpredictable nature of migraines can leave sufferers feeling isolated and helpless at times, potentially spiraling into a state of mental fatigue. When each day comes with the possibility of debilitating pain, the frustration and disappointment can accumulate, sometimes leading to feelings of sadness and depression. It's crucial for those affected to appreciate that their emotional health is just as significant as their physical well-being. Managing depression means acknowledging its presence and seeking ways to nurture one's emotional state.

Healthy coping strategies can serve as effective tools in managing both anxiety and depression related to migraines. For starters, engaging in therapeutic activities like journaling can provide an emotional outlet. Writing down thoughts and feelings not only helps expel negativity but also allows for self-reflection and understanding. Another powerful ally in this battle is physical activity. While it's counterintuitive to exercise through pain, regular physical movement is known to boost mood by releasing endorphins that help reduce stress and anxiety.

In addition, practicing mindfulness and meditation can ground the mind and bring a certain level of peace even when chaos threatens. These practices focus on the present moment, promoting a state of calm stability. By anchoring thoughts, mindfulness can diminish the power of anxiety and ensure that depression doesn't gain a foothold. Techniques like deep breathing exercises or guided imagery can further instill calmness and help release emotional tension.

Building a robust support network is another crucial measure. Migraines can be isolating, but they don't have to be a solitary experience. Leaning on family, friends, or support groups provides not only comfort but also insights. Sometimes just knowing others understand and empathize with your struggles can lighten the load. Healthcare professionals can offer additional perspectives and tools tailored to individual needs, such as cognitive-behavioral therapy (CBT), which is effective in modifying negative thought patterns and promoting emotional resilience.

Professional help should never be overlooked, especially when anxiety and depression start disrupting daily life in significant ways. Consulting a mental health professional can unveil personalized treatment methodologies, such as psychotherapy or medication, which are vital in managing more severe mental health conditions. Open communication with healthcare providers ensures that both emotional and physical aspects of migraine care are integrated, ultimately enhancing one's quality of life.

Self-care is essential. The unpredictability of migraines underscores the importance of establishing a consistent routine that integrates stress-reducing practices into daily life. Whether through quiet moments, indulging in hobbies, or practicing yoga, creating a personalized self-care toolkit can significantly impact emotional health. Even small actions, like ensuring adequate sleep and balanced nutrition, contribute meaningfully to overall wellness.

Empowering oneself with knowledge is yet another component of tackling anxiety and depression linked to migraines. Understanding the triggers, both bodily and emotional, helps in devising practical approaches to preempt these issues. A well-informed individual can better articulate their needs and tailor treatments effectively to their lifestyle.

Importantly, addressing anxiety and depression involves breaking the stigma surrounding mental health. Acknowledge the emotional burden of migraines without judgment and create an environment where it's okay to discuss these issues openly. This openness paves the way for informed conversations about mental health, encouraging a culture of empathy and understanding not just within oneself, but also among one's community.

Ultimately, while migraines can be a significant hurdle, they do not define the person enduring them. By actively addressing the emotional components associated with migraines, individuals can foster a well-rounded approach to managing their condition. This holistic focus paves the way for a more fulfilling life, free from the shadows that anxiety and depression cast. With knowledge, support, and effective strategies, those affected by migraines can reclaim control and, bit by bit, reshape their reality into one where hope and health coexist harmoniously.

Seeking Professional Help

In the complex landscape of managing migraines, recognizing when it's time to seek professional help is a pivotal step towards reclaiming your quality of life. While lifestyle changes, dietary adjustments, and stress management strategies are crucial, they might not be enough for everyone. When migraines begin to interfere significantly with daily life despite these efforts, or when the emotional burden becomes too heavy, it's wise to consider enlisting the expertise of healthcare professionals.

Consulting with a professional doesn't mean conceding defeat. On the contrary, it represents an empowering decision to enrich your journey with expert insights and tailored treatment strategies. Specialists, such as neurologists and headache experts, bring a wealth of knowledge about the latest and most effective treatment options. These professionals can help guide you through advanced medical therapies, provide accurate diagnoses, and work alongside you to optimize your migraine management plan.

The first step in seeking help is to have an open conversation with your primary care physician. This initial dialogue can be invaluable in determining the severity of your migraines and the types of care that might be most beneficial. Your primary care provider can offer referrals to specialists who are trained in migraine treatment, ensuring you receive comprehensive and focused care.

The path to professional help often begins with a detailed assessment. During this evaluation, your healthcare provider will take a thorough medical history, considering factors such as frequency, duration, and intensity of your migraine attacks, as well as any patterns in triggers. They may also ask about your family history of headaches and any related health conditions, which can be crucial for tailoring an effective treatment plan.

The relationship with a healthcare provider should be a partnership. Clear and open communication is key to achieving the best outcomes. Discussing your symptoms honestly—no matter how trivial they may seem—enables your provider to have a complete picture of your condition. This transparency helps in crafting a management plan that's not only effective but also aligns with your lifestyle and personal goals.

In some cases, the complexity of migraine management might necessitate a multidisciplinary approach. This could involve collaborating with various healthcare providers, such as psychologists, physical therapists, or dieticians. Each element of this team can address different aspects of your health, providing a holistic approach to treatment. For instance, a psychologist can assist with stress reduction techniques and cognitive behavioral therapy, which have been shown to reduce the frequency and severity of migraines for some individuals.

Pharmacological interventions are often a critical component of professional treatment. For many, medications are a lifeline that offers relief from debilitating pain. The realm of migraine medication is broad, including both preventive and acute treatment options. Preventive medications aim to reduce the frequency of migraines, while acute treatments are designed to alleviate pain during a migraine attack. A healthcare provider can help navigate this landscape, considering factors such as side effects, contraindications, and interactions with other medications you might be taking.

However, medicine is not a one-size-fits-all solution. What works wonders for one person may not be effective for another. Finding the right medication can sometimes be a trial-and-error process, requiring patience and close monitoring. Having a healthcare team committed to this trial can make the experience less daunting, providing assurance that you're moving towards finding a solution that truly works for you.

In addition to medication, there are emerging treatments and technologies that might be suitable for some patients. These include devices like neuromodulation tools, which use electrical or magnetic stimulation to alter brain activity and reduce migraine symptoms. Staying informed about new treatments can be beneficial, and professionals are typically well-versed in the latest research and trends.

Beyond the physiological aspects, mental health professionals also play a critical role. It's not uncommon for individuals with chronic migraines to experience feelings of anxiety or depression. The inescapable pain and disruption to daily life can take a mental toll. Therapists, especially those specializing in chronic pain and health psychology, can help address these emotional challenges through therapy and coping strategies. By supporting mental health, they contribute to the overall improvement of one's quality of life.

The importance of professional support cannot be overstated, but it thrives on proactive engagement from the migraine sufferer. Building a strong support network, trusting in the expertise of professionals, and taking an active role in decision-making can significantly enhance the effectiveness of treatment. The journey may be winding, but with the right professional guidance, it can also be one filled with hope and substantial progress.

Chapter 22:
Nutrition Plans

Creating a nutrition plan tailored for migraine sufferers is like crafting an individualized roadmap to better health and symptom management. A well-balanced meal plan can serve as the cornerstone of an effective migraine management strategy, where each food choice plays a pivotal role in influencing your body's response to potential triggers. By combining strategic meal planning with nutritional supplements, migraine sufferers can not only address deficiencies but also build resilience against unexpected headache episodes. Embracing nutritional awareness encourages a proactive approach, turning what once seemed like a dietary battle into a journey of empowerment and well-being. As you explore new avenues of nutrition, remember the transformative potential of every mindful choice, nurturing not only your body but also fostering a rejuvenated sense of control over your daily experiences.

Creating Balanced Meal Plans

Nutrition plays a crucial role in managing migraines. It's not just about what you eat, but how you structure your meals throughout the day. Creating balanced meal plans can be a powerful tool in reducing migraine frequency and severity. The process involves selecting foods that provide a steady flow of energy, essential nutrients, and avoiding known migraine triggers.

To start, it's important to establish regular eating patterns. Skipping meals or fasting can provoke migraines, so aim to eat at consistent times each day. Begin by incorporating a rich variety of foods, ensuring each meal includes carbohydrates, proteins, and healthy fats. Complex carbohydrates, such as whole grains, vegetables, and fruits, release energy slowly and help maintain stable blood sugar levels. Pair these with lean proteins and healthy fats to create a meal that not only satisfies but sustains energy over several hours.

For breakfast, consider options like oatmeal topped with seeds and fresh berries, or scrambled eggs with spinach and whole-grain toast. At lunch, a mixed salad with legumes, avocado, grilled chicken, or tofu can provide a balanced mix of nutrients. Dinner could consist of brown rice or quinoa paired with fish, turkey, or lentils, alongside steamed vegetables. Snacks such as nuts, yogurt, or hummus with carrot sticks can keep you energized between meals.

Hydration also plays an essential part in migraine prevention. Dehydration is a known trigger, so incorporating plenty of fluids is vital. Water is the best choice, but herbal teas and water-rich foods like cucumbers or watermelon can also contribute to your daily hydration goals.

However, it's not just about including healthy foods; you also need to be mindful of potential triggers. Common food triggers include caffeine, alcohol, aged cheeses, and foods with additives like MSG or nitrates. Understanding your personal triggers can take time and may involve keeping a detailed food journal in conjunction with a migraine diary. This approach can help you identify patterns between what you eat and your migraine episodes.

Moreover, some individuals with migraines may benefit from certain dietary adjustments or focused nutritional plans, such as a low-glycemic or anti-inflammatory diet. A low-glycemic diet, which emphasizes foods that don't cause a rapid spike in blood sugar, can be beneficial for some sufferers. Foods high in magnesium, riboflavin, and omega-3 fatty acids have shown promise in supporting brain health and reducing the likelihood of migraines.

Working with a healthcare provider or nutritionist can be invaluable in crafting a meal plan tailored to your needs. They can offer advice on how to incorporate beneficial nutrients effectively and safely manage any dietary restrictions. A personalized approach ensures that you're not only avoiding potential triggers but also not unnecessarily eliminating foods that contain important nutrients.

It's also essential to introduce changes gradually. Opting for whole, minimally processed foods over time can positively impact your overall wellbeing and migraine management. The goal is to create a sustainable eating pattern that doesn't feel restrictive or stressful, as heightened stress levels themselves can trigger migraines.

Being mindful of portion sizes is also important. Large meals can sometimes exacerbate symptoms, so smaller, more frequent meals might be necessary to maintain balance throughout the day. Eating slowly and savoring each meal can also aid digestion and increase satisfaction.

Achieving a balanced meal plan is a dynamic process. Continued observation and adaptation will be necessary as migraine triggers can evolve over time. Patience and consistency are key. By focusing on creating nutritious, balanced meals, individuals with migraines can not only seek to prevent attacks but also bolster their overall health, leading to improved quality of life.

Finally, remember that while food is part of the puzzle, a holistic approach that also considers lifestyle changes, stress management, and appropriate medical treatments is essential for comprehensive migraine care. Each element complements the others, paving the way for long-term relief and resilience.

Nutritional Supplements

When it comes to managing migraines, nutritional supplements can be incredibly powerful allies. While not a complete replacement for medication, supplements can enhance the body's natural defenses, potentially easing the frequency and intensity of attacks. In recent years, interest in non-pharmaceutical options has surged among migraine sufferers. This growing attention reflects a collective search for holistic and sustainable solutions to an often debilitating condition. Let's dive into the world of supplements and explore how they can fit within a broader nutrition plan designed specifically for migraine management.

Magnesium is one of the most well-researched supplements for migraines. This mineral plays a critical role in numerous bodily functions, including nerve transmission and muscle contraction. Several studies have suggested that magnesium deficiencies may be linked to migraines, making supplementation a logical choice for some individuals. Those who have tested positive for low magnesium levels might find relief when they start incorporating this supplement into their daily regimen. Some forms, such as magnesium oxide, are commonly recommended, but it's best to consult a healthcare provider before starting any new supplement.

In addition to magnesium, *riboflavin* (Vitamin B2) has shown promise as a nutritional supplement for migraine sufferers. Riboflavin helps with energy production in cells, which is crucial as some research suggests mitochondrial dysfunction could be an underlying factor in migraines. A daily dose of riboflavin, often in conjunction with a balanced diet, could potentially reduce the number of migraine attacks. While more research is required, some individuals have reported significant benefits from this simple intervention.

Another supplement worth considering is *Coenzyme Q10* (CoQ10). This antioxidant helps generate energy in cells and protect against oxidative damage. Like riboflavin, CoQ10 might influence mitochondrial processes, which are increasingly linked to migraine pathology. Anecdotal evidence supports its effectiveness, and although it's less studied than magnesium and riboflavin, CoQ10 is often well-tolerated, making it a viable option for further exploration in the quest for migraine relief.

Feverfew and *butterbur* are herbal supplements that have garnered attention for their potential migraine-relief properties. Feverfew has been used for centuries in traditional medicine practices with claims of anti-inflammatory properties. Some modern studies indicate it might reduce the frequency of migraines, though results are mixed. Butterbur, on the other hand, has some evidence supporting its efficacy but has raised safety concerns due to the presence of pyrrolizidine alkaloids, which can be toxic if not removed properly. Those considering butterbur should ensure they choose products that are certified free of these compounds.

The possible impact of *omega-3 fatty acids* cannot be overlooked when discussing nutritional supplements for migraines. Found in fish oil and flaxseed, omega-3s have anti-inflammatory properties that might decrease the severity and duration of migraine attacks. Regular consumption as part of a health-conscious diet or through supplementation can provide systemic support, potentially reducing the systemic inflammation associated with some migraine patterns.

Not all supplements are created equal, and quality matters immensely. It's crucial to source supplements from reputable brands that undergo third-party testing to ensure purity and potency. Selecting supplements devoid of unnecessary fillers and additives minimizes potential adverse reactions, particularly in individuals who are sensitive to certain food components.

Integrating supplements into a comprehensive nutritional plan involves a strategic approach. This plan should complement dietary considerations already in place, yielding a synergistic effect aimed at optimizing health and reducing migraine occurrences. Supplements should not overshadow the importance of consuming a well-rounded diet rich in fresh fruits, vegetables, lean proteins, and whole grains.

As with any health-related interventions, there's an element of trial and error when it comes to supplements. What offers relief for one person may not work for another, underscoring the need for personalized plans developed in collaboration with healthcare providers. It's essential to monitor one's response closely, adjusting dosage, form, and timing as necessary to maximize benefits.

Emerging research continues to highlight exciting developments in the field of migraine management through nutritional supplements. As scientists delve deeper into the intricate mechanisms of migraines, we can expect more targeted and effective supplementation strategies to become available. Meanwhile, individuals are encouraged to engage in informed discussions with healthcare practitioners, staying updated on the latest evidence and best practices.

In conclusion, nutritional supplements hold promise as a valuable tool within a broader migraine management strategy. They blend ancient wisdom with modern scientific inquiry, offering hope to those seeking greener pastures beyond traditional pharmaceutical approaches. When embraced mindfully, supplements can support the body's innate healing capacities, empowering individuals to take proactive steps towards a migraine-free life.

Chapter 23:
Dealing with Chronic Migraine

L iving with chronic migraine is like navigating a storm that never truly passes, yet finding ways to steer through it requires a blend of persistence, adaptation, and informed action. For many, the first step is understanding that chronic migraines are not just frequent headaches but a complex neurological condition involving deep-seated changes in the brain's chemistry. It's crucial to integrate varied long-term management strategies and partner actively with healthcare professionals who understand the intricacies involved. Embracing lifestyle modifications, such as consistent sleep patterns and stress-reduction practices, can create a stable foundation. At the same time, exploring a range of treatment options—both traditional and alternative—empowers individuals to reclaim a sense of autonomy over their bodies. The path to addressing chronic migraines might be fraught with setbacks, but every choice to pursue effective relief is a testament to resilience and hope. The journey is deeply personal, and while the storm may not fully recede, the capacity to weather it becomes a profound testament to the enduring spirit of those who thrive beyond it.

Understanding Chronic Conditions

In the realm of headaches, the term "chronic" distinguishes itself from the occasional. It's a word that signifies persistence and the challenges that come with it. For those grappling with chronic migraines, this word becomes part of their daily vocabulary. Understanding chronic conditions, particularly chronic migraine, isn't just about enduring. It's about comprehending the complexities that declare these migraines as a long-term companion.

Chronic migraines are defined by their frequency: headaches occurring on 15 or more days per month, for at least three consecutive months, where at least eight of those days feature migraine headaches. This definition alone speaks volumes. It's not just about having frequent migraines; it's about living with a constant, underlying tension that might erupt into a full-blown episode at any given time. Thus, it is essential to delve into what makes these chronic conditions tick.

Firstly, chronic conditions like migraines often result from an interplay of genetic, environmental, and lifestyle factors. Genetics can predispose individuals to migraines, but they're not the sole actors in this drama. Environmental factors such as stress, irregular sleep patterns, and dietary habits can all conspire to turn episodic migraines into chronic ones. This complex interplay underscores the importance of a holistic approach in managing migraines—not just addressing symptoms but also understanding and modifying triggers as much as possible.

The brain of a person with chronic migraines responds differently to external stimuli compared to those without migraines. There is a heightened sensitivity, often described as having a hair-trigger response. This sensitivity can lead to an overload of sensory information, making it easier for various triggers to initiate a migraine. Understanding this sensitivity is crucial for those seeking to manage their chronic migraine condition effectively. It's about painting the broader picture, observing patterns, and responding with targeted strategies.

Chronic conditions like migraines remind us of the concept of neuroplasticity—the brain's ability to reorganize itself. While this might sound discouraging, it's quite the opposite. This adaptability implies that with the right interventions, habits that contribute to chronic migraines can be unlearned, or at least reprogrammed, creating room for more favorable responses to stimuli.

Moreover, chronic migraines often coexist with other health issues, such as anxiety and depression. This comorbidity can complicate treatment and necessitates a comprehensive approach. Addressing chronic migraines isn't merely about medication; it involves a coordinated plan that considers mental health, lifestyle adjustments, and potentially, therapy. It's an opportunity to seek balance and embrace the notion that treating one condition can positively impact another.

There's also the role of healthcare providers. Building a partnership with a knowledgeable practitioner means more than just receiving medication. It means having someone who can guide you through this labyrinth of triggers, suggest lifestyle adjustments, and provide continuous support as you navigate your chronic condition. It means having an ally who understands that chronic migraines are not just headaches; they're a complex condition with physical, emotional, and psychological implications.

Chronic conditions require patience and perseverance. It's about incremental changes that lead to significant improvements over time. The journey towards managing chronic migraines doesn't have a one-size-fits-all solution. Instead, it demands personalized plans that evolve along with one's understanding of their specific condition. This ongoing process of learning and adapting is empowering—it shifts focus from merely enduring the condition to actively managing it.

Understanding chronic conditions like migraines also involves recognizing the resilience of those who live with them. The strength to wake up each day, uncertain of whether it will be a good day or one dominated by pain, is nothing short of heroic. Chronic migraine sufferers develop coping mechanisms over time that help them navigate life's challenges even when they're not feeling their best. This resilience is a testament to their strength and adaptability.

In essence, understanding chronic conditions is about more than just familiarizing oneself with definitions or statistics. It's about genuinely comprehending the daily battles, the scientific nuances, and the emotional landscape that come with conditions like chronic migraine. As knowledge expands, so does the ability to craft tailored strategies for living life not in spite of, but alongside, chronic migraines. It's a call to action—to dig deeper into understanding, to innovate in treatment and support, and above all, to keep hope alive.

Long-Term Management

Navigating the complexities of chronic migraine involves more than just addressing immediate pain relief; it calls for a sustainable, long-term management strategy. This approach considers lifestyle, preventive measures, and consistent monitoring to minimize the impact of migraines on daily life. Taking control of day-to-day routines can greatly improve the quality of life for migraine sufferers.

One vital aspect of managing chronic migraines over the long term is establishing a robust routine. Regularity in daily activities, such as eating and sleeping schedules, can help stabilize the body's internal clock and reduce the frequency of migraine attacks. This doesn't mean living a life devoid of spontaneity, but rather creating a framework within which your body and mind can thrive. Finding a balance between structure and flexibility is key.

Monitoring and recording migraine patterns play an essential role in long-term management. Keeping a detailed migraine journal allows sufferers to track the frequency and severity of their headaches and identify potential triggers and trends. This exercise, though sometimes tedious, enables a proactive approach. The insights gained from journaling can inform discussions with healthcare providers, leading to more personalized and effective treatment plans.

Stress management is another cornerstone of long-term migraine management. Chronic stress can exacerbate migraine symptoms, making effective stress reduction strategies critical. Stress management can be pursued through various techniques like meditation, mindfulness, and regular physical activity. These methods not only help reduce stress but also provide a mental escape and contribute to overall well-being.

Medication management is another essential piece of the puzzle. Working closely with healthcare providers to find the right medication regimen is crucial. This includes not only finding effective acute treatments for migraine attacks but also assessing preventive medications that can reduce the frequency and severity of episodes. Being informed and active in the discussion about medication, including potential side effects, enables migraine sufferers to make the best possible choices for their health regimen.

Beyond medication and stress management, understanding and managing dietary influences can have long-term benefits. Certain foods and drinks can trigger migraines, and keeping track of these can aid in minimizing their occurrence. However, what triggers a migraine in one person may not necessarily affect another the same way, which makes personal insights from a migraine journal invaluable.

Adopting a holistic lifestyle change is often beneficial, incorporating not only physical but also mental and emotional facets of health. Engaging in regular, manageable physical activity that aligns with personal thresholds can be helpful. Exercise has been shown to release endorphins, the body's natural painkillers, as well as improve mood and reduce stress levels. Developing a consistent exercise routine, even if it begins with gentle walks or yoga, can be empowering.

Another important factor is having a strong support network. Social connections with family, friends, or support groups can provide emotional support and encouragement. They can offer practical help, like recognizing precursors to a migraine and assisting where needed. Effective communication with those around you about your condition fosters empathy and understanding, which can alleviate the emotional burden of chronic migraines.

Incorporating technology can also aid in long-term management strategies. Wearable devices and mobile applications designed for migraine monitoring can provide real-time feedback on potential triggers and stressors, offering reminders for medication, and tracking symptoms. These tools facilitate a more integrated approach to management, empowering sufferers with data-driven insights.

Customized action plans are indispensable for managing migraines in the long term. These plans lay out steps to deal with different stages of a migraine—before, during, and after an episode. Preparing an action plan includes having a ready-to-go kit with medications, hydration options, and other comfort measures tailored to the individual's needs. It helps minimize disruption to everyday life and ensures a quicker return to normalcy.

Lastly, managing expectations and setting realistic goals is paramount. Chronic migraine sufferers may not achieve a complete absence of symptoms, but significant improvement is possible. Regularly reviewing and adjusting goals to reflect progress and set new challenges encourages continual development and adaptation of management strategies.

Overall, the journey of managing chronic migraines is personal and evolves over time. Through a combination of structured routines, proactive health monitoring, stress management, dietary adjustments, medication oversight, and support networks, a life with reduced migraine impact is achievable. It takes commitment and perseverance, but the potential for a richer, more fulfilling life makes it a journey worth embarking upon.

Chapter 24:
Seasonal Triggers

Seasonal shifts can craft a symphony of migraine challenges, each with unique rhythms that demand our attention and adaptation. For many, the budding blossoms of spring or the fiery colors of autumn signal more than just a change in scenery; they're harbingers of potential migraine flare-ups. Understanding how these transitions affect your sensitivities can be empowering. Whether it's the barometric pressure fluctuations of a stormy summer or the air's dryness during winter, these changes can ignite a cycle of symptoms you might dread. But knowledge is your ally. By tracking seasonal patterns with mindfulness and adjusting daily routines, such as hydration and air quality control, you can mitigate their impacts. Embracing strategies that anticipate these shifts ensures you're not taken by surprise, providing you with the tools to face each season with resilience, ready to pursue a life not dominated by migraines but enhanced through foresight and preparation.

Identifying Seasonal Patterns

For many migraine sufferers, the changing of the seasons isn't just a predictable weather phenomenon but a harbinger of potential suffering. Identifying seasonal patterns in migraines can be a critical step towards managing and mitigating their effects. As the seasons transition, so do various environmental factors such as temperature, humidity, and air pressure—all of which can play a significant role in triggering migraines.

The connection between migraines and the weather might seem puzzling at first, but there's a logical explanation rooted deeply in human biology. Our bodies are sensitive to environmental changes, and these fluctuations can affect our biological rhythms. For some, this means headaches and migraines at certain times of the year. Consider this: as winter approaches, the days become shorter, and the exposure to natural light ceases to stimulate our brain as it should, sometimes leading to cases of seasonal affective disorder, mood alterations, or worsened migraine episodes.

On the other hand, spring, with its sudden atmospheric changes and frequent precipitation, brings its own set of challenges. A spike in barometric pressure or an unexpected drop can prompt a migraine attack in those who are susceptible. Recognizing these kinds of patterns isn't about just observing the calendar; it's about understanding how your body responds to the endless cycle of seasons.

For some migraine sufferers, the onset of warmer weather in summer or the crisp air of fall triggers specific symptoms. In the summer, the intense sunlight and heat waves can be problematic. Overexposure to the sun's rays without proper protection might not just cause dehydration but can act as a direct migraine trigger. Similarly, fall introduces potential allergens like mold or different pollen that can also intensify migraine episodes for many individuals.

The challenge lies in accurately identifying which of these seasonal variables might be affecting you. Some individuals benefit from documenting their symptoms in a migraine journal, recording the times and conditions under which migraines occur. Over time, patterns may emerge that can help pinpoint whether there is a seasonal trigger at play. Cross-referencing this data with weather reports can also illuminate specific meteorological conditions that coincide with migraine onset.

Simply put, if you notice a consistent correlation between your migraine flare-ups and the time of year, you could be someone who is sensitive to seasonal triggers. A strategic approach includes planning ahead for these times, perhaps by adjusting your lifestyle, revisiting your migraine management plan, or consulting with healthcare providers for tailored advice.

Understanding these seasonal influences empowers sufferers to anticipate potential triggers and make informed decisions. Effective coping mechanisms might involve using sun protection during summer months or employing humidifiers during the dry spells of winter. By preparing and responding to environmental changes, you can take charge of your migraine management.

Incorporating strategies such as staying hydrated, maintaining a consistent sleep schedule, and practicing stress-reduction techniques can also play pivotal roles. They not only contribute to overall wellbeing but significantly mitigate the seasonal impact on migraines. These approaches work hand-in-hand to protect against potential triggers, ultimately aiming for fewer migraine days as the seasons change.

The critical takeaway is that you've got the power to manage your response to these environmental changes.Identify the patterns unique to your situation to develop insights, fostering a nuanced understanding of your condition's intricacies. In doing so, you're not only better equipped to manage migraines but also improve your overall quality of life.

For many, the mere act of acknowledging that migraines are influenced by seasonal patterns can be empowering. It provides a tangible element to focus on, amidst a condition often characterized by its unpredictable nature. This acknowledgment forms the foundation upon which effective prevention and management strategies can be built.

In conclusion, embracing the challenge of identifying seasonal patterns allows migraine sufferers to actively participate in their treatment. The journey towards understanding is personal and might require patience, yet it's this very journey that leads to effective management and, ultimately, a reduction in migraine frequency and severity. As this process unfolds, each discovery becomes a step toward empowerment, illuminating the path toward better health and a more controlled environment.

Adjusting Routines

For many people living with migraines, seasonal shifts can feel like riding a turbulent wave. As temperatures rise or fall, and daylight hours stretch or contract, our bodies respond in myriad ways, often stirring up the intensity of migraines. Embracing these changes and adjusting your routines accordingly can make a significant difference in managing symptoms.

Winter invites us into a world where daylight is scarce, and cold winds brew tension not just in the atmosphere but also in our muscles. It's a perfect time to rethink your daily schedule. Consider aligning your activities with natural light, harnessing its power to boost mood and regulate the body's internal clock. If possible, engage in morning walks to soak up precious sunlight. And if getting outside isn't feasible, a light therapy box may offer a glimmer of relief from those winter blues.

As winter melts into spring, new allergens creep into the air. Flowers bloom, but so do various triggers in pollen form, which can exacerbate migraine episodes. During these months, keep an eye on local pollen forecasts and plan indoor activities on high-pollen days.

An investment in a high-efficiency particulate air (HEPA) filter might prove beneficial in keeping your home free from irritants.

Summer days unfold with intense heat—another notorious migraine trigger. It's a season that calls for meticulous planning and hydration. Your routine might need to be shuffled to include frequent breaks from the sun and adjusting the time of outdoor activities to cooler parts of the day, such as the early mornings or late afternoons. Staying hydrated is crucial; placing reminders throughout your day can keep water intake consistent. A summer hat and a reusable water bottle are more than just accessories; they're essential tools in your migraine management arsenal.

Autumn paints the landscape in colors that are warm yet the air becomes crisp and cool, bringing relief for some, but for others, fall allergies and shifts in barometric pressure can play havoc with migraine cycles. This season encourages us to adapt our routines in preparation for the colder months. Incorporating grounding activities like yoga or tai chi can offer physical comfort, easing tension and promoting relaxation. Warm herbal teas may not only soothe but also provide an opportunity for mindfulness, a moment of pause in our over-scheduled lives.

The transition from one season to another also often means a change in daily habits. Not everyone experiences fatigue in the same way or at the same times; acknowledging your body's signals and adjusting your sleep patterns accordingly can have great payoffs. Small tweaks, like ensuring curtains block early morning sunlight or adjusting the thermostat to night-friendly temperatures, can help align your circadian rhythm.

Fluctuations in weather and temperatures mean fluctuations in our bodies. Each season brings its own set of challenges and, equally, opportunities for improvement. Embracing change, rather than resisting it, empowers migraine sufferers to take command of their health journey. By making calculated adjustments, one can seek a balance that mitigates the impact of migraines. It's about finding that sweet spot in your routine where the mind and body harmonize with nature's rhythm.

Navigating the nuances of seasonal triggers can be daunting, but it also serves as a reminder that empowerment lies in adaptability. Remember, these changes need not happen overnight. Slowly integrating adjustments can make the transition more comfortable and sustainable. Observing how your body responds allows you to refine these practices over time.

Soon, you'll find that these seasonal adjustments aren't just about managing migraines; they're about enhancing your overall well-being. It's about creating a lifestyle resilient enough to weather the unpredictabilities of each season. Embrace the ebb and flow, and your routine becomes a sanctuary—a foundation upon which a healthier, more balanced life is built.

Chapter 25:
Patient Stories and Case Studies

Imagine stepping into the shoes of those who have bravely navigated the labyrinth of migraines, where each story unfolds a unique tapestry of trials and triumphs. These patient stories and case studies don't just illuminate the nuanced realities of living with migraines, but they also offer profound lessons and insights born from personal battles. From discovering unexpected triggers to mastering personalized coping strategies, each narrative serves as both a beacon of hope and a wellspring of wisdom for others on similar journeys. As you delve into these accounts, you'll find that hope often thrives in community and shared experience, lighting the path toward effective management and an improved quality of life. There's something powerfully human about these stories—they remind us that while migraines might be a common adversary, the journeys through them are deeply individual yet remarkably interconnected through shared resilience and understanding.

Personal Accounts

Every migraine story is unique, yet interconnected by a web of shared experiences and challenges. These personal accounts provide a glimpse into the lives of individuals navigating the labyrinth of pain and uncertainty that migraines often inflict. While the clinical definition remains consistent, the lived experience of a migraine can differ dramatically from one person to another, colored by lifestyle, triggers, and the very personal impact on daily life.

Among these stories is that of Emily, a 35-year-old mother of two who began experiencing migraines in her late twenties. Initially, the spasms of light and throbbing pain were sporadic, hitting once every few months. Over the years, they intensified in both frequency and severity. "It was like a shadow, always lurking," she recalls. When Emily speaks of her first debilitating migraine attack, you can sense the fear it incited. What started as a typical day unraveled into one spent in a dark room, blinds drawn, as she battled nausea and blinding pain. Her children learned to tiptoe and communicate through whispers, adapting their lives to the unpredictable rhythms of their mother's condition.

John's journey into the world of migraines took a slightly different path. At 42, he discovered his trigger was less about physiological factors and more about the environment. High-stress corporate meetings, combined with fluorescent lighting, often served as the harbinger for his migraines. "It got to the point where I could predict them as surely as if I'd scheduled them myself," he notes with a touch of humor. He recounts a particularly poignant incident: seated in a boardroom, a presentation looming, when the familiar aura clouded his vision. The pressing need to maintain professionalism while grappling with intensifying pain is a tightrope he learned to walk with some difficulty.

Then there's Kelly, whose adolescence was overshadowed by migraines that few acknowledged due to her young age. Chronic migraines are a cruel visitor for a teenager, she admits, describing the isolation it bred. Missing out on school dances, being absent from pivotal sports events, and the unsympathetic stares from peers who couldn't comprehend her predicament were equally hurting as the migraines themselves. "It felt," she reflects, "like I was always an observer, never a participant." Yet, this pain honed resilience and self-awareness, attributes she carried into adulthood and used as tools for advocacy, offering mentorship to younger migraine sufferers.

The personal account of Rajeev offers another layer to this tapestry of experiences. Migraines didn't strike until after his migration to a new country—a stressful transition compounded by dietary changes and climate variations. In every pounding beat of his migraine, he heard echoes of homesickness and cultural shock. Navigating a healthcare system unfamiliar to him posed its own set of challenges, making the battle against migraines not just physical but deeply cultural as well. His gradual approach to melding traditional remedies with Western pharmacology has brought some relief, though he acknowledges it's an ongoing journey.

Perhaps one of the most heart-wrenching stories is that of Anne, whose migraines painted each stroke of her academic career into a struggle of epic proportions. With aspirations of becoming a neurosurgeon, she found herself perpetually at odds with the brainiac enigma that is a migraine. "It's ironic, in a dark way," she muses, "to study something that's simultaneously sabotaging your efforts." Dual hurdles of workload and frequent absences made her journey arduous, yet, in this crucible of pain and ambition, she found avenues to channel her frustration into research, hoping to unlock answers that eluded her own grasp.

From chaos sprang community for Bianca, whose encounters with migraines drew her towards advocacy. She transformed her personal experiences into a cause, leveraging social media platforms to connect with others and raise awareness about this neurological condition that's often misunderstood. Bianca's approach hinges on support and educating through storytelling, a virtual sanctuary where people gather, recognizing their stories in others and finding solace in shared strategies and victories.

Each story speaks not just of challenges endured, but of resilience rediscovered in unexpected places. Dr. Samir, a healthcare professional who juggles his dedication to his patients with personal battles against migraines, exemplifies this. "Being on both sides of the stethoscope," he explains, "creates a unique empathy. It humbles you, as both healer and patient." His experience serves as a reminder of the intricate relationship between personal experience and professional empathy in healthcare.

These narratives collectively amplify the notion that while migraines can be excruciatingly isolating, sharing these stories dismantles those solitary walls. Personal accounts hold the strength of connection—encouraging others to seek individualized remedies while underscoring a collective understanding. It's this balance of personal struggle and communal support that helps individuals like Rachel, a high school senior who uses her artistic talents to illustrate the 'invisible' nature of migraines, elevating awareness through art.

Through these stories, we see more than just the presence of migraines; we see perseverance, adaptation, and in many cases, transformation. They challenge the misconception that a migraine is merely a headache, enlightening that its impact reaches far beyond the physical, affecting every echelon of a person's life. By delving into these personal accounts, we hope to awaken empathy, inspire strength, and remind each migraine sufferer they're not alone in their journey.

Lessons Learned

Over the course of navigating the complex world of migraines through patient stories and case studies, several illuminating lessons emerge, each offering valuable insights that resonate deeply. These lessons don't just enrich our understanding; they empower those living with migraines by transforming stories into sources of strength and guidance. Each narrative shared has threads of commonality that weave a tapestry of wisdom, revealing truths that aren't just theoretical but lived and felt.

First and foremost, the critical role of self-awareness cannot be understated. Many patients recount the profound impact of understanding their own bodies—learning to read even the subtlest of signals. This awareness becomes a cornerstone in managing migraines, as it helps in pre-empting full-blown episodes. By analyzing triggers and responses, individuals can tailor their environments and routines to better accommodate their unique needs.

Equally significant is the power of adaptability. Migraine sufferers often find themselves presented with unexpected challenges that require flexibility and resilience. Adjusting plans or routines might not initially seem like a formidable strategy, but the adaptability it fosters is a powerful tool in mitigating the frequency and intensity of migraines. This involves everything from tweaking sleep schedules to modifying daily diets to embrace more beneficial nutrients.

Community support emerges as another crucial element. For many, sharing experiences with fellow sufferers provides not just solace, but also practical advice. These shared narratives create a sense of belonging and understanding that is often absent in isolated journeys. The compassion and empathy found in support groups—whether online or in-person—can be incredibly healing, helping sufferers feel less alone in their struggles.

Another profound lesson gleaned from these stories is the importance of comprehensive care. Many find that effective migraine management requires an interdisciplinary approach that spans medication, lifestyle changes, alternative therapies, and mental health support. Working closely with healthcare professionals across fields is critical, as each expert contributes unique insights that can collectively enhance overall well-being.

Personalization also plays a pivotal role. No two migraine experiences are exactly alike, making it essential for individuals to develop personalized strategies. This personalization extends to everything from pinpointing specific dietary triggers to identifying stress management techniques that resonate personally. The emphasis is always on finding what uniquely suits each individual, driving home the point that what works for one might not work for another.

Moreover, embracing patience and perseverance emerges as a recurring theme. Navigating the journey of migraine management is rarely a straight path. It's often fraught with setbacks and disappointments. Yet, the stories highlight that patience—with oneself and with the process—is integral. Persevering despite these setbacks, and celebrating small victories along the way, builds resilience and ultimate success in managing the condition.

Building effective communication bridges cannot be overlooked. Many case studies emphasize the importance of clear and open dialogue—not just with healthcare providers, but with friends, family, and employers. This communication can foster a more supportive environment and reduce misunderstandings, helping those around the sufferer become allies in their management journey.

Perhaps most inspiring is the recurring theme of finding empowerment through education. Knowledge truly is power, and the more individuals learn about their condition, the more capable they become in making informed decisions. Learning about the science of migraines, understanding medical options, and being aware of new research developments instills confidence and a sense of control.

Finally, the stories underscore the transformative power of optimism. Maintaining a positive outlook, even when faced with chronic pain, significantly impacts one's quality of life. This optimism isn't naïve; rather, it serves as a foundation for resilience. It fuels the search for solutions and inspires individuals to keep seeking better outcomes, reminding them that while migraines are a part of their lives, they don't have to define them.

The lessons shared here not only highlight the collective wisdom found in patient stories but also serve as guideposts for anyone navigating the stormy seas of migraines. They remind us that while the journey might be challenging, it's also full of opportunities for growth and empowerment.

Conclusion

As we've journeyed through the intricate landscape of migraines, it's clear that understanding and managing this condition is no small feat. Yet, it's also evident that empowerment through knowledge and practical tools is both attainable and transformative. For those grappling with migraines, life often feels like a delicate balancing act—a continuous quest for equilibrium amidst an unpredictable storm. However, with each chapter of this book, you've been equipped with insights and strategies that illuminate the path toward that balance.

The first step in overcoming any challenge is understanding it. By delving into the science behind migraines and identifying personal triggers, you lay the groundwork for effective management. This understanding provides the very foundation upon which all other strategies are built. Recognizing symptoms and working closely with healthcare providers enhance your capacity to navigate the complexities of diagnosis and treatment. The trust established within a healthcare team becomes a pillar of support, offering guidance and reassurance in moments of need.

Lifestyle adjustments play a pivotal role as well. From crafting a daily routine to ensuring restorative sleep, the changes you implement have the power to ripple through every aspect of your life. These refinements, although sometimes challenging to adopt, offer immense benefits, setting the stage for improved well-being. Nutrition intertwines closely with lifestyle, emphasizing the importance of both avoiding certain foods and embracing beneficial nutrients. Through mindful dietary choices, you not only alleviate symptoms but also cultivate a nurturing relationship with your body.

Stress is an unavoidable part of life, but your response to it can be finely tuned. The stress management techniques discussed empower you to meet life's hurdles with resilience. By incorporating relaxation practices, mindfulness, and meditation, you create a sanctuary of calm amidst chaos. Exercise, too, becomes a cornerstone of well-being, with physical activity tailored to your unique needs providing both physical and mental upliftment.

As you explore medical treatments, it's essential to balance traditional and alternative approaches. With options ranging from over-the-counter medications to prescription solutions, as well as alternative therapies like acupuncture and herbal supplements, you craft a personalized treatment regimen. This holistic approach acknowledges the uniqueness of your migraine experience and respects it with tailored interventions.

Coping strategies further empower you to manage pain and foster emotional resilience. Beyond physical discomfort, migraines can impact emotional well-being, but with strategies for emotional support, you're never in this alone. Journaling offers a reflective space to track patterns and analyze triggers, providing clarity and actionable insights that bring your journey full circle.

Community and communication are integral. Building a support network and enhancing communication with healthcare teams ensure that you're surrounded by understanding and compassion. Navigating social and workplace settings with awareness and forethought creates an environment conducive to your needs, reducing the likelihood of triggers and facilitating understanding from those around you.

Your journey doesn't end here. Whether facing hormonal changes, seasonal triggers, or other unique challenges, continuous adaptation is necessary. Migraine devices and technology offer modern solutions for monitoring and symptom management, while patient stories remind us of the strength in shared experiences. Remember, each person's migraine story is unique, but there is comfort in knowing others walk similar paths.

The insights shared in this book serve as a comprehensive guide meant to empower, inspire, and provide actionable steps towards improving quality of life. Though migraines may remain a part of your story, they do not dictate its entirety. Embrace the strategies, stay informed, and forge a path that aligns with your personal journey. Your empowerment is the ultimate goal, and in that pursuit, know you're supported every step of the way.

Appendix A:
Appendix

In the journey to conquer migraines, knowledge is power. This appendix is crafted to be your steadfast companion, offering a treasure trove of resources and support organizations that can arm you with additional information and guidance. Explore the carefully selected readings to deepen your understanding and discover new perspectives on managing migraines. Connect with a network of support organizations that provide assistance, advocacy, and community for those affected. This appendix isn't just a list—it's an invitation to expand your arsenal of tools, empowering you to take charge of your health and improve your quality of life. By leveraging these resources, you're one step closer to navigating your migraine journey with confidence and clarity.

Resources for Further Reading

In your journey to better understand and manage migraines, having access to a wealth of well-curated resources can play a pivotal role. Knowledge is not only empowering, but it also provides a clearer view of the path to easing the burden of migraines, whether that's through medical, dietary, or lifestyle changes, or simply in finding solace and support. Below, you will find a selection of books, articles, and websites that serve as a compass to navigate the multifaceted world of migraines.

One essential book to consider is "Migraine" by Oliver Sacks. His comprehensive exploration of the neurophysiological aspects of migraines provides illuminating insights into the ways these headaches influence the brain's functioning. With his characteristic blend of neurological expertise and compassionate storytelling, Sacks offers a narrative that is both informative and deeply human.

Another insightful read is "A Brain Wider Than the Sky" by Andrew Levy, which chronicles the author's own battle with migraines. Levy's narrative is compelling due to its candid and often humorous reflection on living with chronic pain. His journey will resonate with anyone who has experienced the life-altering presence of migraines, providing both validation and hope.

For those interested in the psychological and social dimensions of migraines, "Not Tonight: Migraine and the Politics of Gender and Health" by Joanna Kempner offers a provocative examination of how gender impacts perceptions and treatments of migraines. Kempner's work dissects the stigmatization of migraines and uncovers societal biases that have influenced migraine research and policy.

If you're seeking scientific articles that delve into the latest research and treatment options, exploring databases like PubMed can be incredibly valuable. Search for topics like "novel migraine therapies" or "migraine preventive treatments" to find peer-reviewed journals that offer evidence-based insights. Regular access to such journals can keep you abreast of cutting-edge developments and breakthroughs in migraine research.

Online resources, such as the American Migraine Foundation website, provide a wealth of information on all aspects of migraine care, from treatment to patient advocacy. The site is regularly updated with educational articles, webinars, and tips tailored for migraineurs, making it an indispensable resource for ongoing learning.

In the realm of dietary considerations as they relate to migraines, the book "Heal Your Headache: The 1-2-3 Program for Taking Charge of Your Pain" by Dr. David Buchholz is a must-read. Dr. Buchholz presents an actionable approach to identifying and managing dietary triggers, which can be pivotal in reducing the frequency and severity of migraine attacks.

Migraine.com is another excellent online resource. This community-centric platform offers articles, personal stories, and expert advice. It's also a hub for a community of people who understand the impact of chronic migraines, offering both practical tips and emotional support.

In understanding the correlation between lifestyle and migraines, resources that focus on mindfulness and stress management can be vital. "The Mindful Way Workbook" by John Teasdale, Mark Williams, and Zindel Segal is a practical guide to applying mindfulness methods, highlighting techniques to reduce stress and its compounding effect on migraine occurrences.

Don't overlook the role of support organizations, which often provide more than just information. They serve as an essential community where you can find empathy and understanding. The Migraine Trust and the National Headache Foundation are similar in their missions. They aim to improve the lives of those who suffer by promoting awareness, education, and advocacy.

Lastly, for those keen on exploring the intersection of migraines with modern tech, resources that discuss wearable technology and apps for migraine management, like the book "The Wired Body: An Exploration of How Wearable Technology Can Transform Our Lives" by Ned Turner, offers fascinating insights on integrating technology into migraine management strategies.

Collectively, these resources offer an array of perspectives, from scientific to personal. They are invaluable tools in painting a complete picture of migraines, aiding in the demystification of this complex condition. By engaging with these texts and platforms, sufferers and their loved ones can take the first steps towards understanding, managing, and ultimately finding solace in the face of chronic migraines.

Support Organizations

Finding a community that understands what you're going through can be incredibly empowering, especially when dealing with the challenges of migraines. Support organizations play a crucial role in offering both practical advice and emotional support. They provide a safe space where individuals can connect, share experiences, and learn from one another. It's not just about receiving help—it's also about giving it, which can be beneficial for those involved.

One of the most well-known organizations is the American Migraine Foundation. Founded by experts in the field, it's dedicated to improving the lives of people with migraines through research, education, and partnership. They offer a wealth of resources, including a comprehensive list of treatments and coping strategies. Engaging with their community can provide a sense of belonging, knowing that others are walking a similar path.

The Migraine Research Foundation takes a slightly different approach, focusing heavily on funding innovative research to find a cure for migraines. Their efforts have supported numerous studies, breakthroughs, and advancements in understanding the complexities of migraine disorders. Aiding them through donations or participating in fundraising events can be a rewarding way to contribute to the future of migraine research.

Beyond national organizations, local support groups often offer a personalized touch. These groups can bring together people from the same community, fostering not only discussions but also friendships that extend beyond the shared experience of migraines. Meetings can be in-person or virtual, making it easier for people to connect, regardless of their location or physical limitations.

Support organizations also serve as educational hubs. They host workshops and webinars aimed at equipping members with skills to manage their symptoms more effectively. From navigating the healthcare system to finding reliable information about medications, they cover a broad array of topics that can be especially useful for those newly diagnosed. These educational efforts can empower sufferers, enabling them to take control of their own health.

Internationally, organizations like the World Headache Society work towards global awareness. They focus on disseminating knowledge and research across borders, acknowledging the universal experience of migraines while respecting cultural differences in treatment and perception. In these efforts, they highlight the importance of understanding migraines as a worldwide health issue, demanding a unified approach.

An intriguing aspect of participating in these organizations is the advocacy work. Many support groups, both large and small, engage in advocacy efforts to increase public awareness and influence policy related to migraine care. Those interested in advocacy can find numerous opportunities to get involved, from letter-writing campaigns to meetups with legislators, to ensure that migraine sufferers receive the attention and resources they deserve.

In the digital age, online forums and social media groups dedicated to migraines provide another layer of support. While not formal organizations in the traditional sense, they are invaluable for immediate and continuous interaction. Members can post questions, share personal milestones, and simply vent in a space where they feel understood. The convenience and availability of these platforms make them a popular choice for many.

It's important to note that support organizations are just as beneficial for caregivers and loved ones. Understanding the daily struggles faced by someone with migraines can be difficult, but these organizations offer them insights and tools to move from being passive bystanders to active participants in the healing journey. Inclusion in such communities fosters patience and empathy, qualities essential to supporting a person with migraines.

Finding the right support organization can be life-changing. Whether you're drawn to a local group, an international body, or an online forum, the key is engagement. Like any other aspect of managing migraines, involvement in these organizations can help steer the course from feeling isolated to feeling empowered. In this sense, the true value of support lies not just in what you receive, but in what you contribute and how you connect with others.

Finally, remember that the landscape of support organizations is diverse and dynamic. New groups frequently emerge, offering fresh perspectives and innovative approaches. Keeping an open mind and exploring different options can reveal paths that might not have seemed possible before. The right organization for you is out there, waiting to welcome you into its supportive embrace.

Glossary of Terms

This glossary is designed to clarify key terms you'll encounter throughout the journey of managing migraines and related conditions. Understanding these terms can empower you with the language needed to effectively communicate your experiences and work towards improved health and quality of life.

Aura: A set of sensory disturbances experienced before a migraine. They may include visual changes, such as seeing flashing lights or zigzag patterns, as well as sensory changes like tingling in the arms or legs.

Biofeedback: A technique that teaches individuals to control certain bodily functions, such as heart rate or muscle tension, to alleviate migraine symptoms.

Chronic Migraine: A condition characterized by headaches occurring on 15 or more days per month for more than three months, where at least eight days per month have features of a migraine.

Cluster Headache: A severe headache that occurs in cyclical patterns or clusters. It is one of the most painful types of headache.

Comorbidities: Conditions or diseases that occur simultaneously with migraines, such as anxiety, depression, or fibromyalgia.

Botox (OnabotulinumtoxinA): An injectable neurotoxin that can be used as a preventive treatment for chronic migraines.

Electromyography (EMG): A diagnostic procedure to assess the health of muscles and the nerve cells that control them, sometimes used in migraine assessment.

Magnesium: A mineral often recommended as a supplement for some people with migraines due to its potential to alleviate symptoms.

Neurostimulation: A treatment method involving electrical impulses to specific body parts to relieve pain or other symptoms.

Photophobia: Increased sensitivity to light, a common symptom experienced during migraine attacks.

Prodrome: Early symptoms that signal the onset of a migraine, which can include mood changes, neck stiffness, increased thirst, and yawning.

Serotonin: A neurotransmitter believed to play a role in regulating mood, pain, and migraines.

Trigeminal Nerve: The largest cranial nerve that transmits sensory information and can play a significant role in headache disorders, including migraines.

Vestibular Migraine: A type of migraine that involves vertigo or balance issues, often without the classic headache phase.

Visual Snow: A visual disturbance that resembles static or "snow," which can accompany a migraine or occur on its own.

As you continue your exploration of migraine management, refer to this glossary to ground yourself in the essential terms that will aid in understanding and discussing various aspects of this condition.

www.ingramcontent.com/pod-product-compliance
Lightning Source LLC
Chambersburg PA
CBHW020417290526
45785CB00002B/606